HOUSEHOLD
COST OF ILLNESS

HOUSEHOLD COST OF ILLNESS

A Study of Chikungunya Fever

B. P. Chandramohan

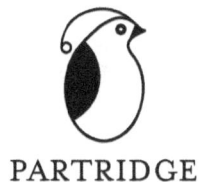

PARTRIDGE

ISBN:	Hardcover	978-1-4828-7124-1
	Softcover	978-1-4828-7123-4
	eBook	978-1-4828-7125-8

Print information available on the last page.

To order additional copies of this book, contact
Partridge India
000 800 10062 62
orders.india@partridgepublishing.com

www.partridgepublishing.com/india

CONTENTS

LIST OF TABLES

LIST OF FIGURES

LIST OF CHARTS/MAPS

Foreword

A basic question that should prompt readers to this book is, "Why should economists worry about *chickungunya*? Is this not an epidemiological problem, and as such, a concern for doctors, medical professionals and public-health officials?"

The author makes a good case to assure us, that disease-analysis need not be restricted to the purview of life sciences alone. Indeed, economics and related disciplines have much to offer public policy in the field of public health management. Consequently, the basic question posed above can be answered in many interesting ways. For instance, he notes from his detailed research that, the economic effects of *chikungunya* are important because the effects reflect the public-health conditions in India. The effect of the disease on people of all ages is quite immense. It is very serious for children, as it leads to increased absenteeism from school. The impact of the disease is also damaging in the case of women, who are pregnant, since there is a substantial increase of miscarriages, still-births and underweight babies. The health effects in the case of adult victims are related to opportunity cost of time and money, which include the explicit cost on cure and the implicit cost due to weakness, morbidity and disability. Hence, *chikungunya* cannot be treated as a pure public-health issue, but should be studied under a framework that relates economic development to infectious diseases and epidemics. Obviously, the disease has also generated negative spillover effects at the national level, in production, tourism and trade. Hence, the book serves a very important purpose, because, the research investigates the economic effects of infectious diseases as these directly affect productivity, nutrition, socio-economic stability and the exacerbation of poverty. The focus of the study is on the economic costs of households managing *chikungunya*, and will be useful for public health policy towards intervention and cure.

It is important to note that the term "Economic Development" covers various issues besides poverty and inequalities of income, thanks to the monumental works by the Nobel Laureate Professor Amartya Sen in *Development as Freedom* Sen explores the relationship between freedom and development, and the ways in which "freedom" is both a basic constituent of development in itself, and an enabling key to other aspects. The usual approach to development is to tie increases in per-capita GDP with overall well-being of a nation. However, Sen suggests that development should be broader, and focus instead on "capabilities" which are "substantive human freedoms". Sen has argued that "capability deprivation" is a better measure of poverty than low income, because it can capture aspects of poverty hidden by income measures. Examples of "capability deprivation" include differences between the US and Europe in healthcare and mortality, comparisons between sub-Saharan Africa and India in literacy and infant mortality, and issues covering gender inequality and "missing women". Most importantly, Sen's works have begun to contest the efficiency of markets, and their ability to provide *public* goods, and has opened up new venues for public policy.

Indeed, one of the most relevant examples of this approach to development has been in the field of public-health management in less-developed economies. Until recently, public-health officials viewed disease control and prevention as purely epidemiological problems. But it has now become clear that public-health management must incorporate epidemiological concerns within the overarching belt of capabilities. For example, The WHO reports that malaria causes over 300 million episodes of "acute illness", and more than one million deaths annually. Most of the deaths occur in poor countries, and especially in sub-Saharan Africa.

In a very important research paper, Gollin and Zimmermann find that ecological differences associated with malaria account for why some countries today are rich and others poor. Indeed, Gallup and Sachs show that countries with intensive malaria had income levels in 1995 only 33% of countries without malaria, whether or not the countries were in Africa. They note that countries that have eliminated malaria in the past half century have all been either subtropical or islands. Interestingly, these countries' economic growth in the five years after eliminating malaria has usually been substantially higher than growth in the neighboring countries. Similarly, Papageorgiou and other researchers connect diseases to economic development find that if infectious diseases are particularly virulent or debilitating, then growth-or development-traps are highly likely. This finding has major implications for cost-effective intervention programs, alongside growth-oriented macroeconomics policies. Another important concern often expressed in these contexts is, "Can markets not efficiently tackle the problem of disease control?" This is also a decent concern, since many fair-minded supporters of market-mechanism, view intervention programs as an excuse for big government. One cannot simply wave away these concerns, as merely extreme positions. Research has to clearly inform us as to whether markets can allocate optimal resources to eradicate diseases and ensure optimal development. Indeed, economists Gersovitz, Malaneyand Berndt, from the World Bank, have measured the viability of markets and the role of externalities to this issue. These researchers have examined the role of government intervention in disease prevention, vaccination, testing and therapy, and in recent years, the issue of "advanced market commitments" for drug procurements and cost effectiveness of disease eradication have been measured to address HIV/AIDS, malaria, and tuberculosis. If people recover to be susceptible, then government action should equally favor both prevention and therapy.

In this context, India provides an excellent case study because, recently, India has undertaken a historic economic reforms program towards liberalization. The capabilities approach to disease prevention and development is appropriate for modeling public health concerns, under such regulatory-induced distortions. That is, moving from central planning towards the price system creates internal costs of adjustments, forcing shadow value of inputs to deviate from their market prices. The approach undertaken by the author in this book is ideal for modeling the hidden costs of diseases.

Another basic question that is usually asked in this context is, "What is the Indian experience in this regard? Are things seriously bad in public-health and is our management and control widely off-target?" This is also interesting questions that question the relevance of any such research project. Interestingly, researchers Panicker and Rajagopalan, Dasgupta, Chow and others find that health improvements in India, while significant, have not kept up with rapid economic growth rates. The poor in India face high out-of-pocket payments for health care, a significant burden of infectious diseases.

Planned increases in public spending will involve making difficult decisions about the most effective and efficient health interventions if they are to translate into improved population health. Results from previous research indicate that India has great potential for improving the health of its people by devoting just one percent of GDP ($6 billion) to a well-designed health program nationwide, which would save nearly 480 million healthy years of life annually. Likewise, in the Indian context, research also shows that there are positive long-term effects of state-sponsored malaria eradication programs on school and educational attainments. Researchers DeLeire and Manning point out that if such illness is prevalent, the effects on labor market equilibrium wage rates could be substantial.

What can we say about Indian experience with chikununya the author notes that the initial episodes of this disease were in Calcutta (July-August 1963) and in Vellore, Tamil Nadu (July–November 1964). These two incidences of *chikungunya* were unnoticed, but a major epidemic of was reported recently during December of 2005 in the twin cities of Hyderabad and Secundarabad, in Andra Pradesh. Since then, India has been facing major outbreaks in various states in following sequence: Karnataka (2005), Maharastra (March, 2006), Orissa (2006) and again Karnataka, Tamil Nadu and Andhra Pradesh (2006), and finally, in Kerala (2007).

In addition, *chikungunya* also attacked Madhya Pradesh, Maharashtra, Gujarat, and Rajasthan. There were 2 million cases in 2006 and an equal number in 2007, which many researchers feel is a highly underreported figure. Social activists and the press portrayed *chikungunya*as the 'greatest neglected disease'. Indeed, during its peak, the disease was more rampant than malaria and dengue.

These recent attacks have suddenly increased public's awareness of the disease, and public health officials have begun to educate themselves and investigate preventive measures. The severity of the problem begged the Union Health Minister to call for an emergency meeting with the health ministers of nine states to discuss preventive measures. Most importantly, the problem highlights the impact of a debilitating infection in working populations, belonging to the low socio-economic background. This is particularly true with *chikungunya* because, the tests are costly, and the National Institute of Virology, Pune, is the only diagnostic centre. Consequently, there is no uniformity in the treatment addressed by medical practitioners in different parts of the country.

Finally, the government of Kerala, for the first time in public health circles, officially confirmed 125 deaths attributed to the disease. The general consensus is that the virus affects immunity. Most patients find it difficult to perform their daily tasks, and they regain their ability to resume work only after a long interval.

Because pure-biological considerations imposed stringent restrictions on policy implications, researchers have begun to develop epidemiological-economic models in the field of public health, such as *Willingness-to-Pay* (WTP) methods. Professor Chandramohan's research contributes to this line of enquiry in two major notable ways. First, it has relevance for the "capabilities" approach and links that approach to second-generation models of *stated preference approach* for India. In that sense, it is the first study of its kind for India. Second, this study is very interesting because of it has collected detailed household-level data from a costal district in India. Such data has never been applied to examine this issue. Extant work on public health and health economics has concentrated on the effects of malaria and similar health concerns. However, the importance of newer strands of viral infections has not been thoroughly integrated into research, and the role of opportunity costs has not been studied within the capabilities framework. Therefore, the author's CV model to test the importance of capabilities and COI of *chikungunya* for India is a significant accomplishment.

S.N. Gajanan
Professor in the Economics department at
University of Pittsburgh at Bradford, Bradford, USA

Preface

C hikungunya fever is a vector –borne disease transmitted by mosquitoes that became widely prevalent in most of the coastal States of Indian Union since 2006. It causes numerous health problems to the victims and cognitive problems for medical practitioners and policy makers. Several episodes of the fever have shown long term physical and neurological disability besides short term morbidity. There is no vaccine available to prevent Chikungunya though it is generally considered non-fatal. Hence the disease can be treated at relatively low cost by simple measures to prevent the severity of the disease. However, poor people treated the diseases relatively costly.

Though the disease was not new to India, the disease caused panic among the public and resulted in socio political and medical concern when the epidemic outbreak penetrated fast in to rural and urban areas after 2006.The symptoms, side effects and socio-economic impacts were not similar in the affected areas. In the Kanyakumari District of Tamil Nadu, the disease inflicted more among the rural agricultural laborers and tapper workers in rubber plantations, resulted in severe loss of employment and productivity. The present study is an attempt to analyse the economic impact of Chikungunya fever at the household level in Kanyakuramari District.

This report presents the results of the study "The Economic Impact of Chikungunya Fever on Household level in Tamil Nadu: A study in Kanyakurmari District" This project is undertaken with the financial support from Malcolm and Elizabeth Adiseshaiah Trust, Chennai. This financial assistance is gratefully acknowledged. I am indebted to Presidency College for providing the necessary facilities to undertake the project. I fail in my duty if I don't mention the helps extended by the post graduate students of Marthandam Christian College, Kanyakumari.

I am indebted to Prof. R.Nagaraj of MIDS for his valuable guidance in undertaking the project. I also gratefully acknowledge the support of Mr.K.Sampath Kumar.

B.P.Chandramohan

Abbreviations

APSED	-	Asia Pacific Strategy for Emerging Diseases
CD	-	Chronic Diseases
CDC	-	Center for Disease Control
CDR	-	Child Death Ratio
CDS	-	Department of Communicable Diseases.
CHC	-	Community Health Center
CHD	-	Coronary Heart Disease
CHIK	-	Chikungunya
COD	-	Cause of Death
COI	-	Cost of Illness
COMBI	-	Communication for Behavioral Impact
CSR	-	Communicable Diseases Surveillance and Response
DALE	-	Disability Adjusted Life Expectancy
DALY	-	Disability Adjusted Life Years
DHC	-	Direct Health Care
DNHC	-	Direct Non-health care costs
ECOC	-	European Center for Disease Control
ELISA	-	Enzyme Linked Immunosorbent Assay
FCM	-	Friction Cost Methods
GBD	-	Global Burden of disease
HALF	-	Health Adjusted Life Expectancy
HQ	-	Head Quarters
IBS	-	Incidence Based Studies
IEC	-	Information Education and communication
IHR	-	International Health Regulation
INHC	-	Indirect Non-health Care Costs
IVM	-	Integrated Vector Management
MRHS	-	Medical & Rural Health Services

NCD	-	Non-Communicable Diseases
NFD	-	Non Fatal Disease
NSAID	-	Non Steroidal Anti Inflammatory Agent
NSS	-	National Sample Survey
NVBDCP	-	National Vector Borne Disease Control Programmes
OOP	-	Out of Pocket
PAF	-	Population Attributable Friction
PAR	-	Population Attributable Risk
PBS	-	Prevalence Based Studies
PCR	-	Polymerase Chain Reaction
PCTS	-	Perspective of Cost of Illness Estimated
PHC	-	Primary Health Center
QALYs	-	Quality Adjusted Life Years
RNA	-	Ribo Nucleic acid virus
RTPCR	-	Reverse Transcriptase Polymerase Chain Reaction
TNMSC	-	Tamil Nadu Medical Service Corporation
UNDP	-	United Nations Development Programme
VBD	-	Vector Borne Diseases
WTP	-	Willingness to Pay
YLD	-	Years Lived with Disability
YLL	-	Years of life lost

Introduction

Mosquitoes are well known as industrious carriers of many infectious diseases such as Malaria, urban Filariasis, and Dengue, Yellow fever, Japanese encephalitis and Chikungunya. Widespread poverty, tropical climate, environmental disturbance such as floods, and a lack of public health infrastructure are some of the important factors that contribute to viral infections through uncontrolled mosquito breeding. Recent research in the economics of epidemiology have evaluated the economic costs of Malaria and Japanese Encephalitis (Gersovitz, 2000; Berndt, 2007; Epstein, 2006; Chow, et al., 2007) and have related these costs to development activities, human interferences, climate changes, ability of parasitic load in the community and socio-cultural practices (Panicker, et.al., 1986; Musgrove, 2004; Juana, et al., 2004; Lindelow, 2005).

Chikungunya is a type of viral fever caused by a single stranded RNA virus of the genus alpha virus in the family of Togaviridae, and the virus is transmitted to humans by the bite of the Aedes aegypti mosquito (Enserink, 2006)[1]. The genus alpha virus had its origin in Africa and it is endemic in rural areas of Africa. It was first described by Marion Robinson and W.H.R. Lumsden in 1995, following the outbreak on the Makonde Plateau, bordering Mozambique in 1952 (Robinson, 1955).

The Aedes aegypti Chikungunya virus transmission cycle has entered Asia where it poses great health problems. The virus is not a stranger to India. It had caused two major outbreaks; in Calcutta, July - August 1963 and in Vellore, July – November 1964 (Shaw et al. 1964). These two incidences of Chikungunya were unnoticed, but a major epidemic of Chikungunya was reported recently during November - December of 2005 in the twin cities of Hyderabad and Secundarabad, in Andhra Pradesh. Since then India has been facing major outbreak of the disease in various States in the following

---

[1.] The name Chikungunya is derived from 'Makonde' - an African Language - which means "bend up", in reference to the stooped posture which develops as a result of arthritic symptoms of the disease.

1

sequence: Karnataka (2005), Maharashtra (March, 2006), Orissa (2006) and again Karnataka and Andhra Pradesh (2006). In 2006, new cases of Chikungunya were reported in Chennai and Salem districts of Tamil Nadu, and finally in the Kanyakumari district of Tamil Nadu and Kerala in 2007. In addition to these four Southern States, Chikungunya also attacked Madhya Pradesh, Maharashtra, Gujarat and Rajasthan[2].

These recent attacks suddenly increased public awareness of the disease, and public health officials began to educate themselves and investigate preventive measures[3]. Most importantly, the problem highlights the impact of a debilitating infection in working populations, belonging to the low socio-economic background. This is particularly true with Chikungunya because, it is difficult to make an accurate diagnosis. Further, the tests are costly, and the National Institute of Virology, Pune, was the only diagnostic centre. Consequently, there was no uniformity in the treatment addressed by medical practitioners in different parts of the country.

The symptoms of Chikungunya are acute infections heralded by fever and severe arthralgia, followed by other constitutional symptoms and rash that may last up to 7 days. The arthralgias affect the small joints of hands, wrists, ankles and feet with lesser involvement of larger joints. Besides pain and swelling, patients may suffer from headaches, photophobia, retro orbital pain and sleepless nights.

Until recently, the scientific literature did not confirm any death, or neuroinvasive effects and hemorrhagic cases related to Chikungunya. However, the government of Kerala, for the first time in public health circles, officially confirmed 125 deaths attributed to the disease. The general consensus, up to this point is that the virus affects immunity. Most patients find it difficult to perform their daily tasks, and they regain their ability to resume work only after a long interval.

The economic effects of Chikungunya are important because it manifests public-health conditions in India. The effect of it on people of all ages is quite immense. However, it is very serious for children, the aged and

---

2. There were 2 million cases in 2006 and an equal number in 2007. Some of the social activists and the press portrayed Chikungunya as the 'greatest neglected disease'. Indeed, during its peak, the disease was more rampant than Malaria and Dengue. Further, we must note that non-availability of tests underestimates the number of affected population.

3. The severity of the problem begged the Union Health Minister to call for an emergency meeting with the health ministers of nine states to discuss preventive.

pregnant women. It was reported that there were incidences of miscarriages, still-births and underweight babies, and increased absenteeism among school children. The health effects of Chikungunya in the case of adult victims are related to opportunity cost of time and money, which include the explicit cost on cure and the implicit cost due to weakness, morbidity and disability. These factors adversely affect household production, and therefore the gross domestic product. Hence, Chikungunya cannot be treated as a pure public-health issue, but should be studied under a framework that relates economic development to infectious diseases and epidemics. Obviously, the disease has created negative spillover effects at the national level, for tourism and trade (Kent, 2006; Levin,Simon, 2007; Gersovitz, et al., 2004; Roberts, 2006). Indeed, we must investigate the economic effects of infectious diseases as these directly affect productivity, nutrition, socio-economic stability and the exacerbation of poverty. The focus of the study is on the economic costs of households managing Chikungunya.

Objectives of the Study

The specific objective of the study is to assess the economic burden of Chikungunya on household level in Kanyakumari District of Tamil Nadu. The supplementary objectives are:

1. To estimate the cost of illness of Chikungunya affected households in Kanyakumari District of Tamil Nadu.
2. To estimate the imputed cost of recovery after resolving Chikungunya fever at the household level.
3. To assess the implications of Chikungunya fever for the households in Kanyakumari District.

Hypotheses

1. Wage loss of the sick person(s) primarily determines the total cost of illness of the Chikungunya affected households.
2. Socio- economic housing and environmental factors are likely to affect more favourably to the infection of Chikungunya fever among wage earners than non-wage earners.

Research Methodology
Data Sources and Survey Design

Both primary and secondary data have been collected for the study. The economic cost of illness has been estimated from an accounting sense using direct cost of Chikungunya.

The location and severity of Chikungunya are mostly determined by climate such as rainfall and the socio-economic conditions of population. On that basis, the Kanyakumari District of Tamil Nadu has been selected as the area of the study. The secondary data and other relevant information have been obtained from the published materials of the Ministry of Health, Government of India, Government of Tamil Nadu and the records of public and private hospitals.

Primary Data (Field Survey)

The field survey was organised to collect relevant data for the cost estimation. At the micro level, a district based cross-sectional survey of households has been conducted to collect primary data. The population is households with Chikungunya episodes during 2007 in Kanyakumari District. The household is therefore the unit of analysis, because it is an important socio-economic unit and an attack of Chikungunya is a drain on the resources of the household. The survey was in such a way planned to conduct ex-post exercises through recalls.

The structured questionnaire is the main instrument for the collection of primary data from households. The demographic and socio-economic characteristics of the households and direct cost of Chikungunya fever episode to the household inclusive of the out-of pocket expenses are sought through addressing the questionnaire to the respondent households.

Survey Design

The survey is designed as an integration of status based and historical approaches which consisted of collection of data on socio-economic status, activity status and health status, besides eliciting information about the impact of Chikungunya fever on the household.

The household data required for the study were collected from 258 households in Kanyakumari District having taken into consideration of the disease prevalence and accessibility. With the help of the district medical officer, the sample villages have been identified. The population of the Chikungunya affected households in each selected village of the district have been finalised with the help of the inputs supplied by the village health assistants. A screening interview was conducted in each selected village to identify the households, which had experienced Chikungunya disease in the reference year of 2007. The screening interview was aimed at establishing that the reported fever is indeed Chikungunya and it occurred in the reference period based on the protocol of the epidemic. To confirm Chikungunya, the victim or the respondent was asked to describe the illness by mentioning two major symptoms of the disease. In addition to this, any documents supporting Chikungunya fever, if any, were verified.

The district hospital in Kanyakumari District and other important clinics and dispensaries were contacted to get necessary information on the preparedness of these institutions in delivering health services to the Chikungunya victims. Apart from this, various facilities rendered for the Chikungunya epidemic, some interesting episodes in the form of case studies of the victims' were collected.

Characteristics of Kanyakumari District

Kanyakumari is the southern district of Tamil Nadu where rubber and banana plantations are the main breeding ground for mosquitoes. The district experiences both South-West and North-East monsoons. The vegetation is moist. The mean average rain fall is more than the average of the state. These characteristics are favourable for the breeding of mosquitoes.

Method of Analysis

Fever is the clinical hallmark of Chikungunya. Fever can be classified into mild, moderate and severe categories on the basis of pain. Though death due to Chikungunya is comparatively very rare or not officially confirmed the complications of it are extremely common which come under the category of moderate fever. Also the cases of mild form of the fever without treatment are very rare. Since the households have to manage the illness with fevers and severe body pain without any effective drug, the households feel panic that would cost them an additional cost. The transportation cost and opportunity costs of caretakers' time are important components in the total cost of illness to the household. The monetary value of caretakers' time is computed by combining how much time caretakers allocated for caring the Chikungunya patients and the monetary equivalent of the value of caretakers time. Since most of the wage payments are in cash, it is easy to calculate the monetary value of caretakers' time.

The fear of contracting Chikungunya also urges people to protect themselves which incur an additional expense of providing intensive care. The direct cost of illness (COI) due to Chikungunya comprises the expenditure on treatment, medicines, medical tests and transportation.

The household cost of treating Chikungunya is:

$$X = H + I$$

Where H = Household cost of treating Chikungunya
        I = Institutional cost of treating Chikungunya

The household cost is expressed as:

$H = h_1 + h_2 + h_3 + h_4 \ldots \ldots h_n$. 1,2...n represents cost of drugs, fees pay for stay at hospital, consultation, medical tests, transportation cost for patient and caretaker.

The implications of Chikungunya fever for households have been analysed by using multiple regression model. Cost of illness of households has been taken as the criterion variable regressed by several independent variables.

The study aims at an objective assessment of the damages incurred to the households by adopting cost of illness approach. The monetisation of health losses borne by the households reporting Chikungunya provides a useful measure of the implications of the disease at the household level. So the valuation of cost of illness provides both a theoretically acceptable and practicable alternative to the subjective assessment methods. The results of the study are useful for the health department of both States and the Union Government to make policy implications for the infectious disease of Chikungunya.

Chapter Outline

The report of the present study is organised into nine chapters.

The introductory chapter describes the statement of the problem, objectives, hypotheses, methodology and the organization of the study.

Chapter II outlines health delivery system in combating infectious diseases in India. Various limitations of health care sector in India are discussed at length, besides the participation of private and public sector.

Chapter III presents various features of Chikungunya fever and its health consequences in various States of India. It incorporates origin, spread, symptoms, treatment and the etymology of Chikungunya fever.

Climate change, Chikungunya infection and vector management issues are discussed in the Fourth chapter.

Chapter V connotes the estimation of cost of illness (COI) issues and discussed the approaches, the methods, and types of estimating the cost of illness of infection diseases.

The socio-economic, housing and environmental characteristics of Chikungunya affected households in Kanyakumari District of Tamil Nadu are portrayed in the sixth chapter.

Chapter VII furnishes the health conditions and the extent of illness in Chikungunya affected households in Kanyakumari District.

Chapter VIII analyses the cost of illness of Chikungunya fever at the Household level in Kanyakumari District.

The concluding chapter gives the summary of the study besides giving some suggestions.

References

Andreano and Helminiak, 1988, 'Economic, Health and Tropical Disease: A Review in Economics', *Health and Tropical Disease*, University of Philippines School of Economics.

Berndt, Ernst R, 2007,'Advance Market Commitments for Vaccines against Neglected Diseases: Estimating Costs and Effectiveness', *Health Economics*, Vol. 16, issue. 5.

Chow, Jeffrey; Darley, Sarah R; Laxminarayan, Ramananm, 2007, 'Cost-effectiveness of Disease Interventions in India'.

Enserink.M, 2006, 'Massive Outbreak Draws Fresh Attention to Little Known Virus', *Science*, Vol. 311, No.1085.

Epstein, Paul R, 2006, 'Climate Change and Public Health: Focusing on Emerging Infectious Diseases', *Smart Growth and Climate Change: Regional Development, Infrastructure and Adaptation*.

Gersovitz, Mark, 2000, 'A Preface to the Economic Analysis of Disease Transmission', *Australian Economic Papers*, Vol. 39, issue. 1.

Gerspvotz, Mark; Hammer, Jeffrey S., 2004, 'The Economical Control of Infectious Diseases' *Economic Journal*, Vol. 114, issue, 492.

Juana, J. S.; Narayana, N.; Mupimpila, C., 2004,'Estimating Household Expenditure on Malaria Interventions in Western Sierra Leone: A Contingent Valuation Approach' *International Journal of Environment and Development,* Vol. 1, issue. 1.

Kent, Mary M; Yin, Sandra, 2006, 'Controlling Infectious Diseases' *Population Bulletin*, Vol. 61, issue. 2.

Levin, Simon a., 2007, 'Introduction: Infectious Diseases' *Environment and Development Economics,* Vol. 12, issue, 5.

Lindelow, Magnus, 2005, 'The Utilisation of Curative Healthcare in Mozambique: Does Income Matter?' *Journal of African Economies*, Vol. 14, issue, 3.

Malaney Pia, 2003, 'Micro-economic Approaches to Evaluating the Burden of Malaria', *CID working paper,* Harvard, No.99.

Musgrove, Philip, ed., 2004, *'Health economics in development'*.

Panicker, K.N. & Rajagopalan, P.K. 1986, 'Vector Control through Integrated Rural Development', *ICMR Bulletin*, Vol.16, No.1.

Roberts, Jennifer A., ed., 2006, *'The Economics of Infectious Disease'*.

Robinson Marion, 1955, 'An Epidemic of Virus Disease in Southern Province, Tanganyika Territory in 1952-53', *Clinical Features,* **Trans Royal Society,** Vol.1.

Shaw K.V. Gibbs C.J. Jr & Banerjee G. 1964, 'Virological Investigation of Epidemic of Haemorhagic Fever in Calcutta – Isolation of Three Chikungunya Virus', *Indian Journal of Medical Research,* Vol. 52.

Shepard D.S., Ettling, M.B., Brinkmann, U & Sauerborn, R. 1991, 'The Economic Cost of Malaria in Africa', *Tropical Medicine and Parasitology,* Vol.42, No.3.

Health Care Delivery System And Combating Of Infectious Diseases

Introduction

Being healthy and having economic security are the basic goals of any individual in a society. Amartya Sen asserted that health is among the basic capabilities that gives value to human life. Good health is vital for human development and productivity of human resource. The role of health as an economic engine has recently received substantial attention. The World Health Organisation (WHO) in its report "Macro Economics and Health for Economic Development" stated that investing in health care infrastructure of developing countries is a prerequisite to stimulating economic development. The report concludes that as with the economic well – being of individual households, population with good health is a critical input into poverty reduction, economic growth, and long term economic development at the scale of whole societies.

Limitations of Health Care Sector in India

India's health care structure has an evolutionary history. The first phase (1947-1983) witnessed effective containment of infectious diseases like Malaria, Smallpox, Plague and Cholera and improvement of various health indicators such as mortality and longevity of life. The second phase began with the first National Health Policy of 1983 that encouraged private health care and expanded publicly funded primary health care. The third phase in the new Millennium witnesses a further shift by having the principles of utilising private sector resources for addressing public sector goals, liberalisation of insurance sector and redefining the role of the State from being a provider to a financier and facilitator of health services. Despite several improvements in health care and innovations in the delivery of health care services, the health care system continues to be unaccountable, inadequately equipped and fails to provide access to health to those for want of ability to pay. Villages have no access to medical care facilities when compared to urban and even when they have accessibility, there is no guarantee for them to get minimum sustainable health care facilities. Health care services are grossly inadequate even to meet the needs of some of the ordinary health problems. India lacks infrastructure and management systems to face some of the new diseases found in the recent years.

The failures of health care delivery to the poor and villagers are due to poor governance, lack of strategic vision and unscientific health care management. Governance of health care is difficult because it interconnected with different socio- economic and cultural factors. Different ministries connected to health care are far more complex with no coordination mechanisms among themselves to fulfil some of their common objectives. The distribution of responsibilities among different tires of governments have affected accountability, health governance and functioning of the private sector. Poor management of resources, low funds, irregular supplies and corruption are the ground level factors adversely impacted the public health delivery system. The apathy of trained medical manpower to work in rural areas has become a major reason for the setback of the system. Leadership and governance are essential to plan, manage, monitor and accept the responsibility of decisions taken.

Health care facilities are one of the basic determinants of human-capital formation and human development. Poor utilisation and availability of health care facilities reflects India's poor status in human Development Index rank that it is only 134 among the 182 countries evaluated by the United Nations Development Program (UNDP) in 2009.

In many States of India there are widespread health infrastructure facilities which seem to be non-functional and unresponsive to majority of the population. Majority of the States do not possess the basic medical infrastructural facilities and manpower. Instead of meeting the newer health challenges, the infrastructural facilities show little progress in health delivery. Most of the victims of the communicable diseases like Chikungunya, Malaria and Dengue hail from poor households who find it extremely difficult to purchase private health care services. Even if they purchased private health services, it will have serious impact on the expenditure pattern on other essential items of their household budget. Both in urban and rural areas, majority of the population do not have basic civic amenities. They live in areas proximate to deteriorating environmental conditions, erode their health culture and finally get trapped in the vicious circle of poverty.

Availability of health infrastructure is only a necessary but not sufficient condition to guarantee the delivery of health services. Access to services is an equally important determinant in meeting the healthcare needs of people, especially those in rural areas. Provision of Ambulance facility is a welcome approach to tackle the problem of lack of accessibility. However, Ambulance services to transport the critically serious patients to referral centres are very minimal. Public transportation between PHC and CHC to the District or State hospitals is inadequate and infrequent.

Public and Private Sector Participation in Health Care

The inadequate and unsatisfactory performance of health delivery in the public health sector has led to an unprecedented growth of the private sector, in both primary and secondary health care all over the country. However these facilities concentrate in some of the top metropolitan cities of India. The difficult part of the private sector participation in health care sector is that it generally provides health care facilities at higher costs, though the quality of the services is relatively better.

The pricing of health care services in private sector depends on the size of capital investment, interest rates and prices of other inputs such as labour, technology, rentals etc. Since profit maximisation is the prime objective of the private health care centres, they appoint unqualified and inexperienced doctors and nurses for lower wages. Most of the good public hospitals are located in the urban areas where price of drugs and tests are less, instead of making them access to the poor; it is the not so poor people who consume these services many times more than the poor. There are also some good private hospitals having the capability of providing reasonably good quality of services at affordable prices to the poor. However, due to the increased cost of inputs and services, the cost of health care services could not be reduced to the level of affordability of the affected households.

There is the non-availability of nationally accepted set of standards and quality assurance mechanism for measuring and guaranteeing good quality against bad. In the health sector, patients' perceptions determine health seeking behaviour. With public health providers face chronic shortage of funds, while private providers seeking to save on costs to maximise profits that work against the interest of poor and rural households. The good quality health service in the long run will be more cost-effective in treating diseases without complications. As long as payments are based on fee for every services and every visit then additional investigation brings revenue to the health provider, discourage motivation to ensure quality and hence patients' safety. The non-development of standards and quality assurance will be a barrier for the expansion of social insurance and financial risk protection that adversely affect the poor.

The role of the government is to protect the patient's welfare without allowing them to be the subjects of exploitation. It requires regulations and strict monitoring. The negative outcomes are health providers facing the risk of many litigation, treatment becomes costly for the patient; and corruptions at the hands of the bureaucracy. The objective of regulation therefore is to increase the awareness and create a sense of accountability regarding the quality of patient care.

Private health care markets are encouraged for compensating the falling public investment on health care to the level of its effective demand. However, the main focus of private health care is on profit maximisation and rarely coincides with the public goals of medical care. Nevertheless the private medical sector has gained dominant presence in all the facets of medical system in India. Over 75 percent of the human resources and advanced medical technology, 68 percent of the estimated 15,097 hospitals and 37 percent of 6, 23,819 total beds are in the private sector (NSS 2001- 02) India's health care system has not been progressing on par with its growing economy and infrastructure development. People in general prefer to seek healthcare services from the private sector. Use of public expenditure on health services is mostly for indoor care, governed by the decisions on cost of health care rather than its quality. Even though the scale of operations of the private sector is not exactly known, it is given that private sector accounts for 67 percent of the 30,000 hospitals and 33 percent of the 1,000,000 beds. Also, the private sector accounts for over 60 percent of the 5 million doctors in the country. Most of the services offered by the private sector are for secondary and tertiary care, and not much for preventive healthcare.

Cost of Health Care System

The important factors that determine the cost of health care system are:

1. The nature of drug regime
2. Accessibility and
3. Availability of appropriate technology.

These three factors require regulation and control in order to ensure a reasonable cost to receive a good health care. The other factors determining the cost of health care are as follows.

Availability of Doctors

It is found that as on September 2004, 633108 doctors were registered with different State Medical Councils in India. It gives a doctor population ratio of 1 for 1676 persons in comparison with 249:1, 209:5, 166:5 and 548:9 of Australia, Canada, United Kingdom and the United States of America respectively. Further, the doctor to population ratio in India is biased in favour of urban areas and the remaining areas are underserved, while hilly regions and tribal areas are un-served. Hence India faces serious short-fall of human resources required for health care that indirectly enhances the cost of health care. The proportion of medical expenditure to the GDP is substantially less in almost all the Plans especially after the initiation of Economic Reforms.

Access to Drugs and Medicines

Drugs and medicines constitute a major portion of the out-of pocket (OOP) spending of households on health care. The National Sample Survey 1999-2000 estimated that the share of drugs of OOP is 83 percent for rural India and 77 percent for urban. The share of drugs in the total inpatient treatment in Rural and Urban India accounts for 56 and 47 percentages respectively. However, it is only 10 percent of the overall budget of the Central and State Governments.

The poor quality of public health care forces patients to seek private health care. It has also shown that the utilisation of public health services by the rich is three times more than that of the poor and there is a considerable decline in the utilisation of health care services by the poor (NSS 1986 -87 and 1995-96). The poor availed medical care mostly for primary care. The inequity in the access and distribution of public medical care has been a cause of concern.

Health sector is complex involving several stakeholders, multiple goals, multiple products and different beneficiaries. Some of the areas of concern of the health sectors, their causes and remedial measures are suggested in the Chart 2.1

Chart 2.1: Areas of concern and relevant reform levers for improving the health delivery

Area of Concern	Causes Amenable to Reforms	Relevant reform Levers
Non- availability of staff	Outdated policies & incentive structure Role of Paramedics limited Remote decision-making	Organizational change and policy reforms Empowerment of nurses and paramedical staff Decentralisation
Weak referral system	Lack of integration, Ignorance of referral system	Strengthen communication and transport infrastructure Behavioural change Health Awareness
Poor service delivery	Weak logistics management, Underutilisation of resources	Data based management planning, monitoring, and control Granting autonomy
Funding shortfalls	Absolute shortfall Systematic inefficiencies	Public – Private Partnerships Increasing government health budgets Organisational change
Lack of accountability for quality of care	Obsession with FP targets Low staff motivation, Lack of transparency	Overall Performance of the health system e-Governance

Financing of Public Health

Health is a state subject and it is being financed by tax and non-tax revenue sources. The pay commission implementation and the fiscal consolidation and stress of the State governments reduced the budgetary allocation towards health. Financing of public health determines the effectiveness of service delivery. It is closely linked to the provision of services and the system's ability to achieve the targeted goals. The National Health Account framework revealed that the health expenditure in India during 2001 -02 was approximately Rs. 108732 crore or 4.8 percent of the GDP at the current market price. Out of this, the public spending shares only 1.24 percent of the GDP.

The share of health care expenditure in Revenue expenditure of Tamil Nadu and India is given in Table 2.1.

Table 2.1: Share of health care public expenditure in revenue budget (in percentage)

Years	Tamil Nadu	All States
1985 – 86	7.47	7.02
1991 – 92	4.82	5.72
1995 – 96	6.4	5.7
1999 – 00	5.51	5.48
2003 – 04 (R.E)	5.26	4.97
2004 – 05 (B.E)	4.91	4.71

Source: Compiled from annual budget statements of India and Tamil Nadu.

According to the consumer expenditure data, the percentage share of health care expenditure of households on the total expenditure and non-food expenditure accounts for 6 and 11 respectively. Data also show an increasing growth rate of 14 percent per annum in household health spending; almost half the spending was on outpatient care (52nd Round of NSS).

Public spending on health in India gradually increased from 0.22 percent in 1950- 51 to 1.05 percent during the mid- 1980's and stagnated at around 0.9 percent of the GDP. Estimates show that the per capita expenditure by the government is far below the international average of USD 12 recommended by WDR (WB) and USD 36 recommended by WHO.

The health care expenditure in most of the developing and the all developing countries are higher than India. But a majority of their population has medical insurance hence higher cost of medical expenses do not affect the utilisation of medical facilities. In India, the percentage of people covered under medical insurance is very small. Moreover due to their illiteracy and complexity of availing these facilities there is more difficulty to bring more people under the insurance net. There exist five forms of healthcare insurances- such as private insurance, social insurance, employer-provided cover, community insurance schemes, and government healthcare. It is noteworthy that only 3 to 4 percent of population is insured under in any one of these five insurance forms. However, the insured population has grown to 100 percent in the last 2 years. It is estimated that about 160 million people would be covered by 2010, which is less than 15 percent of the population.

Insurance services without the availability of reasonable quality healthcare services delivery will not serve the intended purpose (Bhat Ramesh, and Saha Somen 2004).

The macroeconomic scenario of Indian Health care sector is not very encouraging. The total annual expenditure on health is around Rs.110, 000 crore, accounting for 5.2 percent of the GDP. However, public health investment on health has declined to 0.9 percent of the GDP by 2001 in comparison with that of the same in China, Sri Lanka and Nepal recording 2, 1.8 and 1.6 percentages respectively of their GDPs. Central Government's contribution to overall public health expenditure by the states is limited to 15 percent. Central budgetary allocation for health has remained static at 1.3 percent of the total central budget. However, budgetary allocations of the States on health have declined from 7 percent to less than 5.5 percent. Decline of public expenditure on health connotes the greater possibility of exclusion of poor from health care facilities. The exclusion of poor from the health care facilities is an important cause of concern. Availability and access to public health facilities is relatively poor for women, children, and the socially disadvantaged sections of the society. The poor performance of public health system in rural areas forces even the poor to seek healthcare facilities from private sector.

There is no close association between per capita public spending and household expenditure. As the actual access depends upon other factors such as the efficiency with which the system is functioning. If the health system is not properly maintained, increase of public expenditure may have little consequence on the improvement of healthcare. Discussions on health care financing in India are centred on the issues of financial constraints of the public sector and the efficiency of resource allocation by the government. Excessive financial burden of households on health reflects frequent use of health care services and greater availability of different types of health practitioners because of the several branches of medicine.

The structure of the State expenditure on health shows that salaries and wage accounts for more than two-thirds followed by medicines, machinery and buildings respectively. The severe crunch of resources forced the state governments to levy user charges for services in hospitals. But it is very cheap for public health care than the private health care. After 1991-92, the proportionate share of public spending of the central government for already financially stressed States shows a gradual reduction. There is a sharp reduction in investment in buildings, sheer increase in disease burden in absolute terms and low priority to preventive and promotion of health.

Health Care Delivery System of Tamil Nadu

Health care is primarily a state subject in India and the responsibility of health delivery rests with the respective State governments. Tamil Nadu has recorded commendable achievements in public health services when compared to the same in other States and Union Territories through the window network of health infrastructure and accessibility to health services. The public health services paid dividend to social infrastructures like literacy, drinking water supply and sanitation and small family norms.

In terms of Human Development Index, Tamil Nadu stands fourth with 0.531 points as against India's average of 0.472 in 2003. Tamil Nadu has achieved considerable success in combating communicable diseases. The Health care infrastructure of Tamil Nadu consists of five types of health care units, viz. Sub-centre, Primary Health Centre (PHC), Community Health Centre (CHC), Dispensaries and Hospitals. The first three categories of health care infrastructure have been designed jointly to address the issue of rural morbidity whereas the last two types cater to the needs of urban health care demand. These institutions are expected to provide collectively the health care objective of preventive, curative and rehabilitative services.

Most of the decline in infant mortality rates has been associated with the control of diarrhoeal disease and respiratory infections, reflecting the expansion of sanitation, immunisation and mother and child services in rural areas. At present there are 1,413 Primary Health Centres including 59 Community Health Centres functioning in the State for rural services.

Primary Health Centres

The PHC is the basic health unit to provide an integrated curative and preventive health care to the rural population with emphasis on preventive and promotional aspects of health care. The national health plan proposed one PHC for every 30,000 rural populations in plains and one PHC for every 20,000 population in hilly, tribal and backward areas.

Utilisation of public health services depends upon the perception of health needs by any community. The location, nature and quality of services are the other associated factors determining the level of utilisation. The behaviour and attitude of service providers also have an impact upon utilisation of health services. The utilisation patterns of both public and private health care services in Tamil Nadu are much better than that of the same in other States, except Kerala.

The differentials in health status among the population in different categories of states in India are shown in Table.2.2. According to the latest health statistics, the Child Death Ratio (CDR) for Tamil Nadu is 7.9; Infant Mortality Rate is 44/1000 live births and the life expectancy at birth is 64.1 years

Table 2.2: Differentials in health status among states

Sector	Population Below BPL (percentage)	IMR 1999-SRS	<5 Mortality (NFHS II)	Weight under3 years	MMR per lakh (Annual Report 2000)
India	**26.1**	**70**	**94.9**	**47**	**408**
Rural	27.09	75	103.7	49.6	-
Urban	23.62	44	63.1	38.4	-
Better Performing States					
Kerala	12.72	14	18.8	27	87
Maharashtra	25.02	48	58.1	50	135
Tamil Nadu	21.12	52	63.3	37	79
Low Performing States					
Orissa	47.15	97	104.4	54	498
Bihar	42.60	63	105.1	54	707
Rajasthan	15.28	81	114.9	51	607
UP	31.15	84	122.5	52	707

Source: SRS and National Family Health Survey

The up-gradation of every district hospital into a medical college hospital ensured the referral need of specialties as well as the steady supply of doctors to work in the rural areas compensating for the migration of doctors to towns, cities and other states as well as overseas. Availability is not a problem but utilisation of such facilities by the people. Tamil Nadu is a good example of a State where health situation has improved significantly in recent years due to the multi-faceted development efforts taken by the government. However, The Government's average contribution to the total healthcare expenditure of an individual is only 20 percent that means out-of-pocket expenditure is as high as 80 percent. On the other hand, the average cost of healthcare has been increasing rapidly. As a result, large majority of the population cannot afford to the rising healthcare expenses.

Tamil Nadu Medical Service Corporation (TNMSC) has implemented an excellent logistics management system to coordinate the activities of purchase, storage, and distribution of drugs and medicines in Tamil Nadu (TNMSC, 2003). It deals with 75 vendors for 600 items for an annual purchase of Rs.120 crores. TNMSC has ensured ready availability of quality drugs and medicines in more than 11,000 government medical institutions throughout the state which includes 9000 sub health centres, 1500 PHCs, 250 Taluk Headquarter hospitals, and 250 veterinary institutions. TNMSC has expended its activities to improve the state of health system in Tamil Nadu by managing a master health check up scheme at the Government general hospital, Chennai; managing the procurement and services of CT-Scans in all district hospitals, managing a special class maternity ward in the Institute of Obstetrics and Gynaecology at Chennai on a very nominal fee fixed by the government, and so on.

Health Care Infrastructure

In Tamil Nadu health services are provided through four directorates, Viz, Directorate of:

1. Medical and Rural Health Services
2. Public Health
3. Indian Medicine and Homeopathy and
4. Family Welfare.

The directorate of family welfare is sponsored by the Central Government and some minor provision is making under State plan. There are some schemes and projects sponsored by foreign agencies like DANIDA (Danish Development Authority). In Tamil Nadu the medical Service Corporation acts as a nodal agency in supplying equipment and medicines to various hospitals. The state has a relatively very good health infrastructure in urban and rural areas. The vital health indicators of Tamil Nadu are shown in Table 2.3.

Table 2.3: Health indicators of Tamil Nadu

Item	Tamil Nadu	India
Crude B.R. (SRS -2008)	16	22.8
Crude D.R.(SRS -2008)	7.4	7.4
Total fertility rate (2008)	1.7	2.6
IMR (2008)	3.1	53
Maternal Mortality Rate (2004-06)	111	254

Source: Registrar General, DPH and PM

Most of the health indicators related to Tamil Nadu is much better than the average of all India. Even at the international comparison, Tamil Nadu was taken as a model State for other underdeveloped regions of the world to follow. However, the infrastructural facilities related to health care are inadequate. The important health infrastructure of Tamil Nadu is shown in Table 2.4.

Table 2.4: Health infrastructure of Tamil Nadu as on, March 2008

Health infrastructure	Required	In Position	Shortfall
Sub- centre	7057	8706	-
Primary health centre	1173	1215	-
Multi- purpose worker (female)	9921	10343	-
Community Health Centre	293	206	87
Health Worker (male)	8706	3278	5428
Health Assistant (female)	1215	1362	-
Health Assistant (Male) at PHCs	1215	303	912
Doctor at PHCs	1215	2260	-
Obstetricians and gynaecologists	206	-	-
Physicians at CHCs	206	-	-
Paediatricians at CHCs	206	-	-
Total specialists at CHCs	824	-	-
Radiographers	206	-	-
Pharmacists	1421	1349	72
Laboratory technicians	1421	909	512
Nurse and Midwife	2657	-	-

Source: RHS Bulletin, March, 2008.

It is interesting to note that some of the components of health infrastructure of Tamil Nadu are more than what is actually required. Only in the cases of community health centre, male health workers seem less than the required level. Availability of health centres and health workers are not sufficient to ensure quality health care. The statistics related to other important health institutions of Tamil Nadu is shown in Table 2.5.

Table 2.5: Other health institutions in Tamil Nadu

Health Institutions	Total Number
Medical college	25
District hospitals	27
Referral hospitals	100
City family welfare centre	104
Rural dispensaries	1421
Ayurvedic hospitals	7
Ayurvedic dispensaries	35
Unani hospitals	1
Unani dispensaries	21
Homeopathy hospitals	9
Homeopathy dispensaries	46

Source: RHS Bulletin, March, 2008.

Medical and Rural Health Services

The Director of Medical and Rural Health Services is in charge of planning and executing of all programmes of Medical Services in Tamil Nadu. The director is responsible for rendering the Medical Care Services through the grid of 29 District Head quarters Hospitals, 152 Taluk Hospitals 80 Non Taluk Hospitals.

The State has been divided into 32 Revenue Districts of the implementation of the Medical Services. The joint Director of Health Services are the overall Controlling officers of all the Medical Institutions for the implementation of Medical Services including family Welfare and supervising authority for all health programmes. The integrated activities of Medical services in Tamil Nadu for long helped to achieve better human development indicators. Table 2.6 shows important indicators of human development in comparison with other states.

Table 2.6: Indicators of human development for major states

Major States	Life expectancy at birth (2002- 2006)			Infant Mortality Rate (per 1000 live births) 2007			Birth rate (per 1000) (2008)	Death rate (per 1000) (2008)
	Male	Female	Total	Male	Female	Total		
Andhra Pradesh	62.9	65.5	64.4	54	55	54	18.4	7.5
Assam	58.6	59.3	58.9	64	67	66	23.9	8.6
Bihar	62.2	60.4	61.6	57	58	58	28.9	7.3
Gujarat	62.9	65.2	64.1	50	54	52	22.6	6.9
Haryana	65.9	66.3	66.2	55	56	55	23.0	6.9
Karnataka	63.6	67.1	65.3	46	47	47	19.8	7.4
Kerala	71.4	76.3	74	12	13	13	14.6	6.6
Madhya Pradesh	58.1	57.9	58	72	72	72	28.0	8.6
Maharashtra	66.0	68.4	67.2	33	35	34	17.9	6.6
Orissa	59.5	59.6	59.6	70	72	71	21.4	9
Punjab	68.4	70.4	69.4	42	45	43	17.3	7.2
Rajasthan	61.5	62.3	62	63	67	65	27.5	6.8
TamilNadu	65.0	67.4	66.2	34	36	35	16.0	7.4
Uttar Pradesh	60.3	59.5	60	67	70	69	29.1	8.4
West Bengal	64.1	65.8	64.9	36	37	37	17.5	6.2
India	62.6	64.2	63.5	55	56	55	22.8	7.4

Source: Sample Registration System, Office of the Registrar General, India, Ministry of Home Affairs.

There are physical, social and economic dimensions of accessibility. Much of the data is available only on physical accessibility such as number of villages which clients' perceptions on access to services record indicators such as travel time to health services, convenience of hours of functioning and availability of health care providers when the facility is available.

Tamil Nadu possesses relatively good quality of health care services especially in maternal and child health care services. The accessibility of health services in Tamil Nadu is good. Majority of its villages and urban centres are located within a half a kilometre travelling distance from a government health care facility. Mere existence of a health facility does not guarantee access to services. Two important reasons for the non-use of government health facilities are distance and inconvenience of timings.

Another important feature of health services in Tamil Nadu is that clinical supplies, equipments and drugs are available in hospitals but not in CHCs and PHCs. Technical competence of personals in rural areas is less than the required levels and motivation of front-line workers is also low.

Health care in a developing country like India is primarily the responsibility of the government. Government involves in health care sector because of providing safety net for the poor, promoting equity and alleviating poverty. Government subsidisation of health care cost is one of the important measures for improving the welfare of the poor. In this framework, basic health can preserve and promote the use of the asset, raising productivity levels and thereby income. The achievement of Tamil Nadu in the demographic front is one of the best next only to Goa and Kerala. According to the India Human Development Report, the general health conditions among women and aged and the short-term health situation in Tamil Nadu is far from satisfactory. Like most of the States, the major provider of primary health care, especially in rural areas is the public sector in Tamil Nadu. The overall performance of health care in Tamil Nadu is reflected in the expected life of a person at birth over a period of time. The expectation of life of birth is shown in Table 2.7.

The statistics show that the expectation of life of both male and female in Tamil Nadu is ahead of the average expected life of male and female at the all India level. It is more pronounced after the 1971 census.

Table 2.7: Expectation of life at birth

Period	Tamil Nadu		India	
	Male	Female	Male	Female
1891-1901	26.21	27.13	23.60	23.96
1901-1911	25.92	27.65	22.59	23.31
1911-1921	19.75	24.23	19.42	20.91
1921-1931	28.71	30.94	26.91	26.56
1931-1941	35.03	36.17	32.09	31.37
1941-1951	36.22	37.23	32.45	31.66
1951-1961	41.09	39.24	41.89	40.55
1961-1971	47.50	46.50	46.40	44.70
1971-1981	52.50	51.90	51.40	50.20
1981-1991	57.40	58.50	55.90	55.90
1991-1996	62.85	63.05	60.60	61.70

1996-2000	63.90	65.90	61.00	62.70
1997-2001	64.10	66.10	61.30	63.00
2001-2005	64.80	67.10	62.30	63.90
2002-2006	65.00	67.40	62.60	64.20

Source: SRS Based Abridged Life Table Sample Registration System, Office of the Registrar General, India.

Figure 2.1: Expectation of life at birth

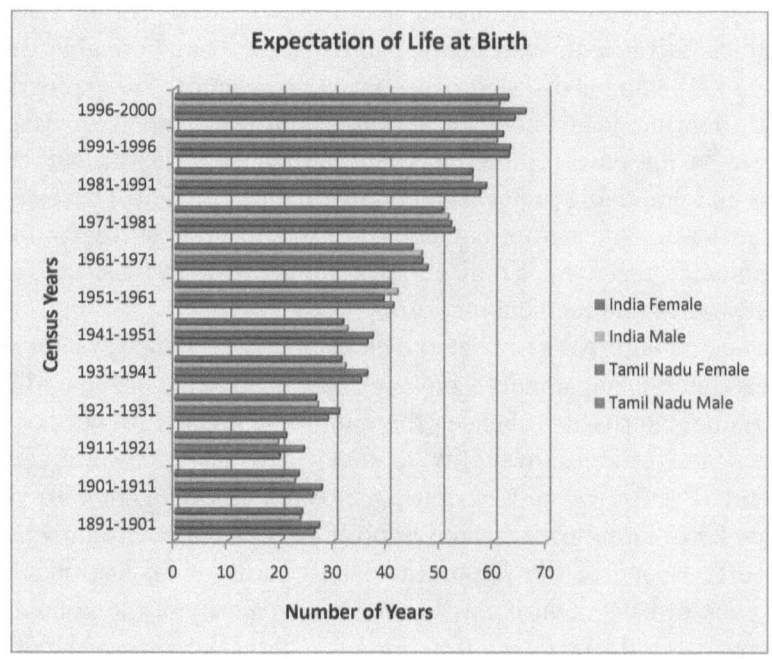

Communicable Diseases

The most common cause of morbidity and mortality among the poor households in developing countries is communicable diseases. The conditions leading to an epidemic are mostly caused by secondary effects, especially by vectors. Communicable diseases refer to diseases that can be transmitted and make people ill. They are caused by infective agents such as bacteria and viruses, which invade and caused damages to the body cells and functions. These infective agents can spread from a source of infection to a person through various routes of transmission. Communicable diseases like Chikungunya, Malaria and Dengue are transmitted through mosquitoes (vector-borne). The infective agents namely virus breed in the body of insects or contaminate the legs and mouths of the insects and infect human when the insects bite humans or by cross-contamination. The hosts refer to the susceptible population. Some people are more prone to become the hosts. Mostly people habitat in a degraded environment, elders with chronic diseases are more susceptible to infection. There are a number of factors crucial to the spread of communicable diseases such as infective agent, source of infection, mode of transmission and the host. They are collectively known as the chain of transmission.

Measures to prevent communicable diseases often prevent epidemics. In addition to preventive measures, most of the communicable diseases require a well planned disaster management programme. These programmes include creating local stock of supplies and equipment for diagnosis, treatment in the case of outbreaks, strengthening of health surveillance systems and practicing protocols for managing information. These are some of the necessary measures but not sufficient to address the problem of communicable diseases. Eradication of communicable diseases requires both preventive and medical measures.

Suspected outbreaks indicated by a health surveillance system need to be investigated using standard protocol. The controlling of the outbreak of a communicable disease reduces the number of cases through preventive activities and reduces mortality due to early detections and effective treatment. Preventive and curative measures work together to prevent infection by isolating patients and improvement of the environment.

Poverty is one of the important determinants of ill-health and vice versa. Lack of basic health care services for majority of the population in the degraded and unhygienic environment, total collapse of health care machinery during the epidemic crisis and population crossed 1.21 billion are some of the stumbling blocks to achieve considerable health care progress in India. Diseases claimed to be under control such as Malaria, Dengue and Chikungunya resurface with renewed vengeance. Dengue was predominantly an urban problem but outbreaks have been reported from rural areas also. The latest problem is the similarity of symptoms of Dengue and Chikungunya diseases in the absence of immediate testing.

Health care is a merit good, generates value to the society above its utility to the private individual. In the case of pure public goods, no one is excluded from consumption as vector control to prevent infectious diseases such as Malaria and Chikungunya fever. Even in the private health care sector, government has an important role to play. Due to asymmetric information, individual consumer of a private medical service is not in a position to evaluate the quality of service; government can guarantee the quality through certification procedures to control these market failures.

Emergence of new communicable disease such as Chikungunya increased the effective demand for more health care facilities and health care providers. The private medical facilities are skewed in favour of urban areas whereas there is acute shortage of trained human resources and medical facilities in rural areas. The health insurance policy no matter how small is the number of holders of such policies gets such services located at a long distance entail huge indirect expenses in the form of loss of wages, transport cost etc. The private hospitals and medical centres are not regulated on the basis of a frame work of rules and hence do not check unethical practices and conflict of social interest. The incidences of fees sharing over prescription of drugs and patients subjected to unnecessary tests. Tamil Nadu achieved good success in combating communicable diseases, Mortality due to communicable diseases has fallen much faster than that of the non-communicable diseases. What the most important for Tamil Nadu is good governance of medical system that facilitates the households to get the best medical care at an affordable cost even to the poor.

References

Arrow, K.J., H.B.Chenery, B.S. Minhas, and R.M.Solow, 1961, 'Capital-Labor Substitution and Economic Efficiency', *Review of Economic Studies,* 43 pp. 225-250.

Athreya Venkatesh and Sheela Rani Chunkath, 1998, 'Gender and Infant Survival in Rural Tamil Nadu: Situation and Strategy' *Economic and Political Weekly.*

Bajpai P.K, 1998, *Social work perspective on Health*, Rawat Publishing, New Delhi.

Baskara Rao N, 1976 *Family Panning in India*, Vikas Publishing House Private Ltd, New Delhi.

Berman Peter, 1995, *Health Sector Reform in Developing Countries. Making Health Development Sustainable*, Harvard University Press, Boston.

Bhat Ramesh and Saha Somen, 2004, 'Health Insurance Not a Panacea', *Economic and Political Weekly*, August 14, pp. 3667-3670.

Bose Ashish, Devenora et al, (ed.), 2002, *Social Statistics, Health and Education*, Vikas Publishing House Private Ltd., New Delhi.

Bradlay D. J, 1993, 'Human Tropical Diseases in a Changing Environment', *CIBA Foundation Symposium*, 175:146-62; Discussion, pp. 162-170.

Bridgman R.F, 1970, *The Rural Hospital; Its Structure and Organization*s, World Health Organisation, Geneva.

Broot G.D, 1938, *Health through Project,* Barnes and Company, New York.

Burton I, R. W Kates and G.F. White, 1993, *The Environment as a Hazard*, Guilford Press, New York.

Casman E.A and H. Dowlatabadi, 2002, *Contextual Determinants of Malaria*, Resources for the Future Press, Washington, D C.

Chalkely A.M, 1986, *A Text Book for the Health workers*, The Christian Literature Society, Madras.

Chan N.Y, Eb K.L, Smith F, Wilson T. F, and, Smith, A.E, 1999, An Integrated Assessment Framework for Climate Change and Infectious Diseases, *Environmental Health Perspectives,* 107, pp. 329-337.

Chauhan Devraj and Sangita Kamdar, 1997, 'Social Sector and Development Focus on Health Care', *Yojana*, Vol.41, No, 4, P.13.

Cll-Mckinsey and Company, 2003, 'Healthcare in India: The Road Ahead', *Ninth Five year Plan: 1997-2002*, Government of India, New Delhi.

Colwell R.R, and Patz J, 1998, *A Climate Infections Disease and Health*, American Academy of Microbiology, Washington D C, USA.

Colwell R.R, 1996, 'Global Climate and Infections Disease: The Cholera Paradigm', *Science,* 274 (5295) pp.2025-2031.

Cooper Michael H. and Antony (ed.),1973, *Health Economics*, Penguin Books Ltd, England.

EpsteinP.R, 1999, 'Climate and health', *Science*, 285 pp. 347-348.

FRCH, 1987, *Health Status of the Indian People: Supplementary Document to Health for All- An Alternative Strategy,* Foundation for Research in Community Health, Bombay.

Government of India, 1999, *Bulletin on Rural Health Statistics in India,* Rural Health Division, Directorate General of Health Services, Ministry of Health and family welfare, New Delhi.

Government of India, 2004, *SRS Bulletin*, Registrar General, New Delhi, India, Vol.38, No.1.

Government of India, *National Sample Survey*, 1986-87 and 1995-96.

Government of India, *National Sample Survey*, 57th Round, 'Survey of Unorganised Services', 2001-02.

Government of Tamil Nadu, 1998, *Economic Appraisal, 1997-98*, P.135.

Gubler D.J et al, 2001, 'Climate Variability and Change in the United States: Potential Impacts on Vector- and Rodent- Borne Diseases,' *Environment Health Perspectives*, 109 Suppl. 2, pp. 223-233.

Harvey D.A, 2005, *Brief History of Neoliberalism,* Oxford University Press, Oxford.

Hetzel B. S, 1980, *The Story of Iodine Deficiency an International Challenge in Nutrition*, Oxford University Press, Oxford.

Imrana Qudeer, 2001, *Public Health and the poverty of Nations*, Vikas Publishing House Pvt, Ltd, New Delhi.

Jackson E K, 1995, 'Climate Change and Global infection Disease Threats', *Medical Journal*, Australia, 163, pp.570-574.

Jetten. T and Focks D, 1997, 'Potential changes in the Distribution of Dengue Transmission under Climate Warming', *American Journal of Tropical Medicine*, 57, pp.285-97.

John H. Bryant, 1998, 'Health for All: The Dream and the Reality', *Health Action,* P.37.

John T J, 2008, 'Resurgence of Diphtheria in the 21 Century', *Indian Journal of Medical Research*, 128, pp.669-70.

John T J, 2009, 'Lessons from the Challenges of Polio Eradication in India', *National Medical Journal of India*, 22 pp.4-8.

John T J, Muliyil J, 2009, 'Public Health is Infrastructure for Human Development', *Indian Journal of Medical Research*, 130, pp.9-11.

Kamali S. S, 1983, Rural *Development and Social change in India*, D.K. Publications, New Delhi.

Karl T.R and Trenbath K, 2003, 'Modern Climate Change', *Science,* 302, pp. 1719-1723.

Kawachi I, Wamale S, (eds.), 2007, *Globalization and Health,* Oxford University Press.

Krasovec Katherine and Show Paul R, 2000, 'Reproductive Health and Health Sector Reform Linking Outcome to Action' *The World Bank*, World Bank Institute, Washington D.C., USA.

Kurusamy S, 1998, 'Planning for Health', *Social welfare*, Vol.38, No.I, P.12.

Lakshmi R. 2003, 'Awareness and Health of Rural woman', *Social Welfare,* vol.4, No.2, P.37.

Lee K, 'Globalization'in Defels R, Beaglehole R, Lansang M A, Gulliford M (eds.), 2009, *Oxford Textbook of Public Health* (5th edn.) Oxford University Press, Oxford.

Lingsay S.W and M.H Birky, 1996, 'Climate Change and Malaria Transmission', *Annals of Tropical medicine and Parasitological*, 90(6), pp. 573-588.

Madiw G, et al, 1997, 'Epidemiology and Treatment of Cyclospora Cayetanensis Infection of Peruvian Children', *Clinical Infectious Diseases,* 24(5), pp. 977-981.

Marten P, 1997, 'Health Impacts of Climate Change and Ozone Depletion: An Eco-Epidemiological medaling Approach', 158.

Mavalankar Dileep, Ramani K.V, Jane Show, 2003, 'Management of R H Services in India and the need for Health System Reform' Working Paper, 09-04, *Indian Institute for Management Association*.

Mc Michael A.J, 2001, *Human Frontiers, Environment and Disease: Past Patterns, Future Uncertainties*, Cambridge University Press, Cambridge.

Metha S.R, 1992, *Society and Health,* Vikas Publishing House Pvt. Ltd, New Delhi.

Millennium Ecosystem Assessment, 2005, *Ecosystems and Human well- being, Synthesis Report*, Washington DC, Island Press,

Nakicenovic N, and R.J Swart, (eds.), 2001, *IPCC Special Report on Emissions Scenarios*, Cambridge University Press, Cambridge.

Nicholls N, 1994, 'El Nino –Southern Oscillation and Vector bone Disease', in *Health and climate change*, (ed.), D. Sharp, Lancet, pp.21-22.

PAHO, 1982, 'Epidemiologic Disease Surveillance after Disaster', *Scientific Publication*, 420, pp. 3-4, and 'Emergency Vector Control after Natural Disaster', *Scientific Publication,* 419.

Park J.E. and Park.K, 1983, 'Health Care of the Community', *Text Book of Preventive and Social Medicine,* Banarsidas, Jabalpur, P.535.

Population Reference Bureau, 2004, *Improving the Health of the World's Poorest People*, Policy Brief, Washington D.C.

Rameshwaran G, 1989, *Medical and Health Administration in Rural India,* Ashish Publishing House, New Delhi, P.18.

Rao R Sujatha, 2004, 'Health Insurance Concepts, Issues and challenges,' *Economic and Political Weekly*, August 21, pp. 3835-3844.

Ratnasamy Prabhavati, 2000, 'Health Care is a Right Not Privilege', *Social Welfare*, Vol.47, No.1, P.33.

Reddy K S, Shah B, Varghese C, Ramada's A, 2005, 'Responding to the Threat of Chronic Diseases in India', *Lancet*, 366, pp.1744-9.

Sachs J.D, 2005, *The End of Poverty: Economic Possibilities for Our Time*, Penguin, New York.

Salazar- Lindo E, Pinell-Salles P, Marcy A, and Chea- woo E,1997, 'El Nino and Diarrhoea and Dehydration in Lima, Peru', *Lancet*, 350 (9091) pp.1597-1598.

Santer and Neun, 1960, *Health Economics*, Irwin Publication, London, P.5.

Santer and Neun, 1996, *Health Economics*, Irwin Publication, London.

Seul S.L, 1975, *Health Administration in India*, Dawn Books, Calcutta.

Shangar Uma and Misra Girish K, (ed) 1993,*Urban health System*, Reliance Publishing House, New Delhi.

Sharp, Ansel M and Register, Charles A, 1987, *Economics of Social Issues,* Universal Book Stall, New Delhi.

Sharp, Ansell M and Register Charles A, 1987, *Economics of Social Issues,*" Universal Book Stall, New Delhi.

Stine R, 1995, 'Global warming if the Mercury Soars, So may Health Hazards'. News and Comments, *Science,* 267 pp. 957-958.

Thaper S. T, 1977, ***Health and Development***, Association of Voluntary Agencies for Rural Development, New Delhi.

The Hindu, 1999, 'Major Health Care Scheme for Poor', ***The Hindu*** Daily, 9 Nov.

Umashankar P.K and Girish K. Misra (ed), 1993, ***Urban Health System***, Reliance Publishing House, New Delhi, P.150.

Verma K.K, 1992, ***Health Care and Family Welfare***, Mittal Publications, New Delhi.

Visaria L, 2000, 'Innovations in Tamil Nadu', Presented at a Symposium on ***The State of our Public Health System***.

Vishwakarma R.K, 1993, ***Health Status of the Under Privileged***, Reliance Publishing House, New Delhi.

Weiss R.A and Michael A. J, 2004, 'Social and Environmental Risk Factors in the Emergence of Infectious Diseases', ***Nature med,*** 10 P.570.

Wilson M L, 2001, 'Ecology and Infections disease' in ***Ecosystem Change and Public Health: A Global Perspective***, Aron J.L. and Patz, J.A, (eds.), John Hopkins University Press, Baltimore, USA, pp.283-324.

World Bank, 1997, The ***State in a Changing World; World Development Report 1997***, Oxford University Press, Oxford.

Features Of Chikungunya Fever And
Its Health Consequences

Introduction

C hikungunya emerged as the major epidemic, a vector-borne disease of considerable importance in India in recent years. Massive and sudden outbreaks of Chikungunya characterising high morbidity rates and prolonged polyrathrities put considerable proportion of the affected population in acute health deficit. The current chapter explains the outbreak of Chikungunya fever and its spread, the epidemiology of the disease, clinical features, diagnosis, treatment and the general socio-economic impact.

Origin

The name Chikungunya is derived from the root verb of Kimakonde language that means "which bends up" or gives stooped appearance of arthralgia. Epidemics resembling Chikungunya fever were recorded in India as early as 1924. However the virus was first spotted in 1952-53, immediately prior to the disease was first described by Marion Robinson and W.H.R. Lumsden in 1955. Chikungunya is believed to have originated in Africa where it has maintained in 'Sylvatic cycle' involving wild primates and forest dwelling mosquito. It was subsequently spread to Asia where it was transmitted through an urban transmission cycle from human to human mainly through by Aedes aegypti mosquito and to a lesser extent by Aedes albopictus. With the same epidemiological profile more outbreaks have occurred subsequently in both Asia and Africa. Outside India, in other Asian countries Chikungunya appeared in Bangkok in 1960s, Indonesia in 1999 and re-emerged in 2005-2006. In various Indian Ocean islands (Comoros, Mauritius, Reunion Islands Seychelles) and in many South East Asian countries including India, the Chik fever reoccurred after a gap of more than

20 years. The Kolkatta outbreak in 1963 started in the south-east monsoon month of July reaching the peak in November and then rapidly declining in December that year. Immediately after that in 1964 Chikungunya affected various parts of India including Vellore and some pockets in the State of Maharashtra. The entry of Chikungunya virus in India is unknown, although Kolkata Sea and air routes were believed to be the problem entry points in India. There were hundreds of cases of Chikungunya during the 1963-64 outbreaks with haemorrhagic manifestations and some deaths. Chikungunya virus had almost disappeared from India after 1973 and since then, no case was reported till the end of 2005.

The Chikungunya virus was first sited in 1952-53, in Tanzania. Chikungunya fever was considered clinically indistinguishable from Dengue and Malaria fever. Genetic analysis reveals that Chikungunya fever originated in tropical forest and subsequently evolved into three distinct, genotypes – the East African, the West African and Asian genotypes. The past outbreaks prior to 2006 were caused by the Asian genotypes. The virus strains currently circulating in India have evolved from East African genotype. Complete information about this disease is not available to the health specialists because of different types of indeterminacies about its causes and spread.

Outbreak

The history of the spread of Chikungunya fever shows that it occurs and then intermittently outbreaks spread to various countries within a short span of time. The spread of the disease is like an epidemic making a sizeable proportion of the population unproductive at least in the short-run. In 2006 in the La Reunion Chikungunya fever was affected by roughly one third of its total population. Based on the empirical literature it is found that the inter-epidemic period of Chikungunya ranges from 4-8 years or as long as 20 years. Outbreaks are most likely to occur in post monsoon period when the vector density is very high. Lack of immunity and inefficient vector control activity in the affected areas are some of the important factors triggering the spread of the disease. Environmental factors and community behaviours also play a significant role in the outbreak and spread of the disease. Major determinant of outbreak dynamics is the ecological cycle of the virus and its vector.

Prevalence in India

Chikungunya fever re-emerged for the first time in Andhra Pradesh subsequently with a series of outbreaks in most of the Coastal States of the rest of the country. As per the data from the National Vector Borne Disease Control Programme (NVBDCP) there were 104 million suspected and 1985 confirmed Chikungunya cases in 2006 to 2008 from 15 States and Union territories. The health system of the country was put into an important test, faced challenges in ensuring timely and rapid availability of standardised drugs, vaccines and diagnostic measures.

Large outbreaks emerged in India in 2006, initially in Andhra Pradesh. The fever then spread to 16 other States infecting more than 1.39 million people. In 2007, 59535 cases were suspected of having Chikungunya fever and in 2008 the provisional figures went up to 71222. The significance of the spread is that new cases have appeared in areas not affected by the epidemic earlier.

Various factors contribute to the outbreak of Chikungunya fever include mutation of the virus, lack of herd immunity and insufficient vector control activity. Urbanisation, migration and increasing population density have significantly contributed to the spread of Chikungunya. Unhygienic environment and improper waste disposal are the other reasons cited for the causes of its spread.

Nearly 10 million people were infected by Chikungunya in the State of Maharashtra alone between 2006 and 2008. Almost all the coastal States of India had many people affected by Chikungunya during the calendar year 2006. Reasons such as lack of budget, lack of medication and limited medical manpower were the reasons for not initiating satisfactory actions to overcome the disease. In most of the State's public health care system was found wanting. Affected people preferred to get access with private medical practitioners rather than the Public Health Centre (PHC) system for health care services. The details of registered cases of Chikungunya in different states are furnished in Table 3.1.

Breeding Areas

Aedes Aegypti mosquito generally breeds in stored fresh water in containers in urban and semi-urban environments. Stagnation of rain water during monsoon in household containers allows breading of Aedes mosquitoes. Aedes Aegyti, the vector mosquito of Chikungunya breeds in man-made containers like cement tanks, overhead tanks, and underground tanks, tyres, coolers, pitchers, discarded containers, coconut shells etc in which water stagnates for more than a week. In the event of improper environmental management, the spread of the disease will become fast and ultimately unmanageable. The disease reoccurs in a seasonal pattern, depending upon the change in climate. The spread of the Chikungunya infection is facilitated by poor hygiene and sanitation conditions and climate change.

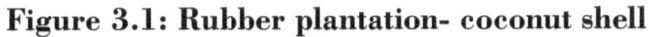

Figure 3.1: Rubber plantation- coconut shell

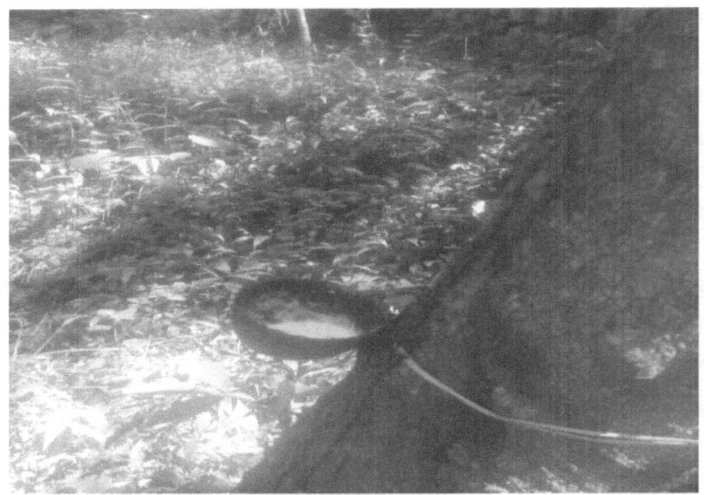

Etymology

Virus

Chikungunya fever is caused by Chik virus that belongs to the Alphavirus genus of the Togaviridae family. It has a single-stranded RNA genome, a 60-70 nanometre diameter capsid and a phospholipids envelope. The virus is mostly found in tropical areas restricted to Asia and Africa. Two distinct lineage of Chikungunya virus could be traced by doing the genetic sequencing of Chikungunya virus. Aedes aegypti remains the major vector in India. Although in some of the affected areas, Aedes albopictus are found in high density. It highlights the capacity of the disease to emerge, re-emerge and spread quickly and also raises questions about factors that can trigger the appearance or the disappearance of the disease. This vector is much more resilient, able to survive in both rural and urban environments, and has a much wider geographical distribution across the world.

The Alpha virus consists of 28 viruses of around 70 nm in diameter. It is characterised by inactivation by diethyl ether or sodium de-oxy chlorate. The complete nucleotide sequences of Chikungunya virus have been determined thrice. The first one was in 1953 of Tanzania strains by Ross and, then in 1983 of Senegal strain and third time in Japan in 2002. Phylogenetic analyses based on partial E1 sequences from African and Asian Isolates revealed the existence of three distinct Chikungunya virus phylogroup; first containing all Isolates from West Africa, second containing isolates from Asia, and third corresponding to East, Central and South African isolates. They have worldwide distribution and all alpha viruses are antigenetically related.

The viruses are inactivated by acid pH, heat, lipid solvent, detergents, bleach, phenol, 70 percent alcohol and formaldehyde. Most of the viruses possess haemog intonating activities. The Chik virus is spherical and consists of an icosahedra capsid surrounded by a tightly adherent lipid envelope covered with glycoproted peplomers. It is a single stranded, positive RNA enveloped virus with a genome size of 11-12kb.

Table 3.1: Number of Chikungunya cases registered

States	2006			2007			2008		
	Total Cases	Samples	Confirmed	Total	Samples	Confirmed	Total	Samples	Confirmed
Andhra Pradesh	77535	1224	248	39	39	11	5	2	1
Karnataka	762026	5000	298	1705	641	133	41227	1442	478
Maharashtra	270116	5901	804	1762	297	135	343	44	19
Tamil Nadu	64812	648	116	45	13	10	3	0	0
Madhya Pradesh	60132	892	106	0	0	0	0	0	0
Gujarat	75419	1155	225	3223	238	122	139	28	3
Kerala	70731	235	43	24052	4732	909	22815	888	220
A & N island	1549	0	0	0	0	0	0	0	0
Delhi	560	560	67	203	203	22	0	0	0
Rajasthan	102	44	24	2	2	2	0	0	0
Pondicherry	542	52	9	0	0	0	0	0	0
Goa	287	75	2	93	93	18	16	14	3
Orissa	6461	171	34	4065	423	90	0	0	0
West Bengal	21	0	21	19138	1135	347	0	0	0
Lakshadweep	35	0	0	5184	10	10	0	0	0
Uttar Pradesh	4	4	4	4	4	4	0	0	0
Haryana	0	0	0	20	20	13	0	0	0
Total	1390322	15961	2001	59535	7850	1826	64548	2418	724

Source: NVBDCP, India

Vectors

The Chik virus is transmitted by culicine mosquitoes such as Aedes aegypti, Aedes albopictus and Aedes Polynesiensis that are commonly involved in the transmission. Culex has also been reported for the transmission in some cases. A recent Indian study reported the transmission of Chikungunya virus by Anopheles stephensi. Chik Virus, Aedes albopictus (Asian tiger mosquito) is considered as the vector for the spread of Chikungunya fever in Indian Ocean Islands. However, Aedes aegypti is the main vector responsible for India. Effective transmission of the virus depends on susceptibility of the vectors, its breading and biting habits and its availability in abundance in the environment.

The physical appearance of the mosquito shows one pair of wings and pair of beams long antennae, a long horn, and a body covered with scales decorated with white or silver plated spots. Other characteristic of the Aedes aegypti mosquito is the Aecles that measure 8 to 10 mm in length. The different species of the Aedes mosquitoes cannot be easily distinguishable by naked eye. Aedes, albopictus is more active outdoors, while Aedes, aegypti feeds and rests indoor.

Figure 3.2: Aedes albopictus

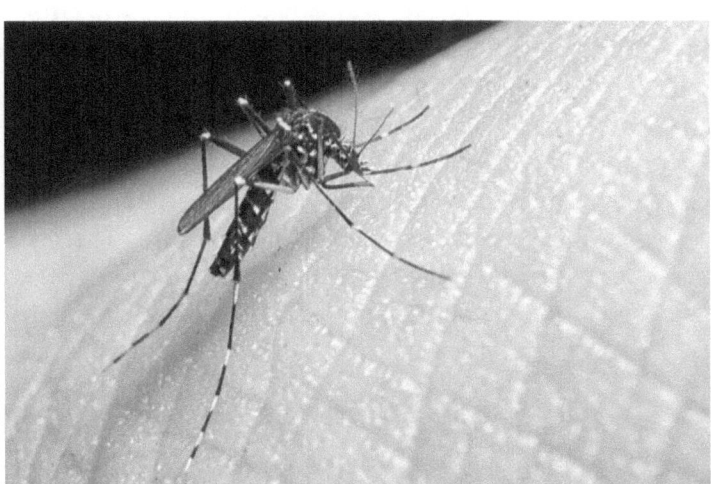

Aedes albopictus, originally indigenous to South East Asia had spread recently in many parts of the world, apparently through carriage of dormant eggs along with transportation of tyres. This is a competent vector for various arboviruses including Chikungunya that has alarmed health authorities for the possible spread of the disease across the world. High virus loads in patients returning from Indian Ocean islands to countries where Aedes albopictus is prevalent might be a source of epidemic in their native countries.

Figure 3.3: Aedes aegypti

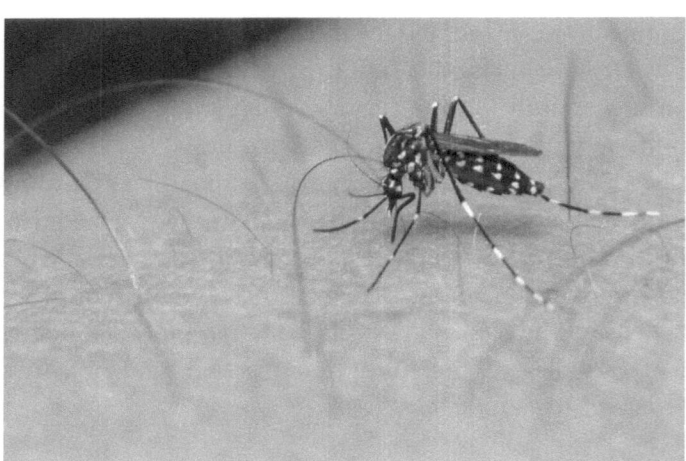

Aedes aegypti is an efficient vector because of its peculiar features like preference for human blood for feeding and have the characteristics of daytime biting habits. Moreover, it is capable of biting several people in a short span of time for one blood meal and the bite is almost painless.

The directorate of public health predicted a high incidence of Chikungunya due to increase in the population of the Aedes mosquito. These mosquitoes cause Ross river disease and Chikungunya. The resurgence of Chikungunya fever in India into viral mutation and emergence of Aedes albopictus is one of the more efficient vectors transmitting the disease.

Figure 3.4: Tiger Mosquito

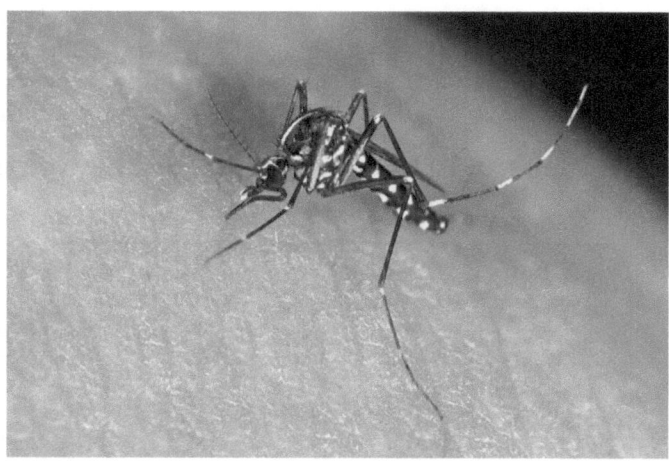

Aedes albopictus was the principal vector in the outbreak of Indian Ocean Islands. Aedes Aegypti in the 2006 Indian epidemic, Anopheles is the predominant circulating vector species in Orissa and Madhya Pradesh and A. albopictus in Tamil Nadu and South East Asia. The most effective vector for human transmission is the predominant species in transmission in animals. Aedes albopictus was readily infected but its transmission was low. In 2007, the outbreak in Kerala, Aedes albopictus played a very important role. It has been proposed that rubber plantations in the state allowed for prolific breeding of this mosquito.

Reservoirs

The common reservoirs for Chikungunya virus are monkeys and other vertebrates. In the current outbreak, suspected reservoirs were macaque monkeys, lemurs and bald mouse. In the epidemic period human beings act as reservoir.

Transmission

Transmission cycles of different geographical genotypes of viruses are different. It is characterised by the circulation periodicity during which disease is transmitted to hosts in silent intervals lasting for about three years during which virus is maintained in primates. In Asian countries

Chikungunya virus transmission is characterised by the absence of an animal and reservoir and direct human to human transmission through peri-domestic mosquitoes.

The agent, host and environment of Chikungunya fever is shown in Chart.3.1.

Chart 3.1: Agent, host and environment of Chikungunya.

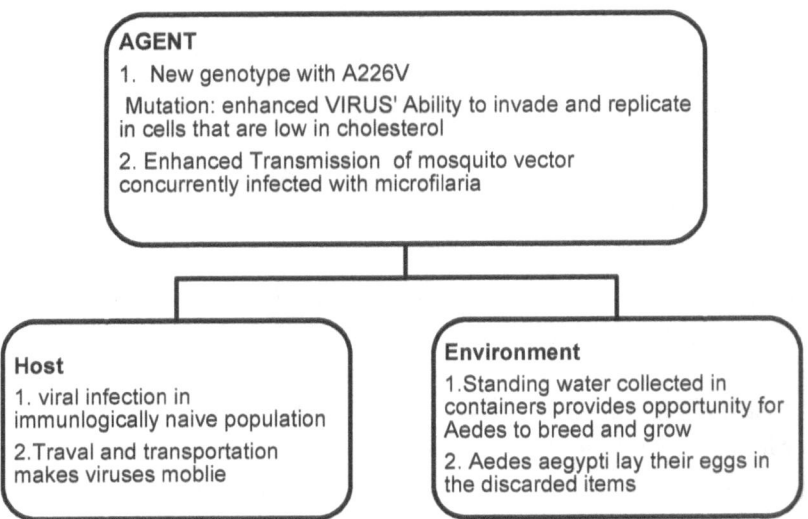

The blood of the affected person contain Chik virus during the "viremic period" or viremia. This period starts on the first day of symptoms and casts until the fifth day. The virus is therefore transmitted from human to the mosquito when a human is bitten by a mosquito during the viremic period. Chart 3.2. shows the man-mosquito–man transmission of Chikungunya fever.

Chart 3.2: Man-Mosquito-Man transmission

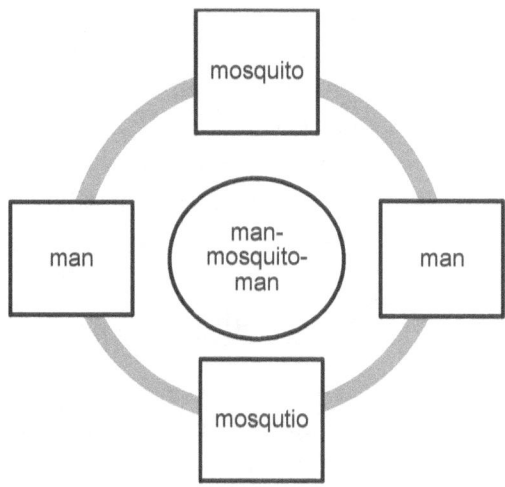

In the past, Chikungunya fever used to be a disease mainly of the tropics until its spread to Italy in 2007 and the subsequent local transmission by the vector, Aedes albopictus.

Among the potential vectors, species of such genus, Aediomorphus, Aedes dalzieli, Aedes vittatus, and Aedes avgenteopunctatus are also thought to be involved in the transmission; the role of cattle and rodents has also been reported in the transmission of the virus. The female mosquito introduces hernoboscis directly into a capillary beneath the skin where saliva containing the virus is injected. The transmission route of the chik virus is furnished in chart 3.3.

Chart 3.3: The transmission route of chik virus.

Lifecycle of Chikungunya Virus

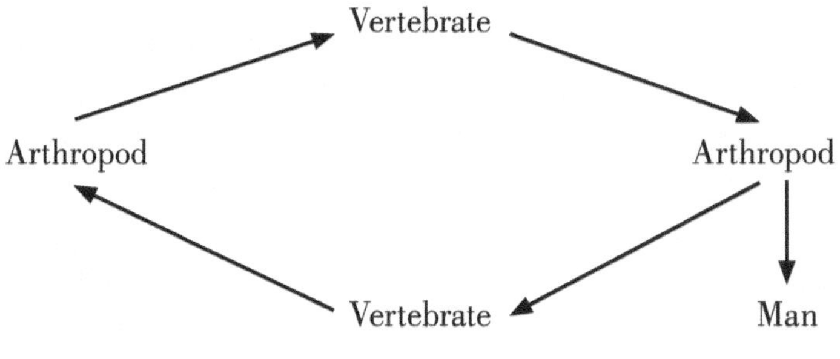

Other modes of transmission include vertical transmission of the virus in mosquitoes by gregarines parasites. The latter has a role in transmission especially during inter-epidemic period. Low level human to human transmission is known in Chikungunya. Due to the resemblance of symptoms to Dengue fever the diagnosis may be missed in inter-epidemic period. This may be responsible for the resurgence of Chikungunya.

Mutation of the virus, absence of herd immunity, lack of vector control and globalization of trade and travel might have contributed to the resurgence of the infection.

Human-Mosquito Human link

Human is the only host serving as reservoir of infection and transmission is sustained by human – mosquito - human cycle through primates. No sylvatic cycle has been reported in Asia as witnessed in Africa, There is no evidence for transovarial (vertical) transmission but co-infection or dual infection with Dengue is possible. Mother to child transmission and co-infection has also been reported recently. This disease is highly infectious and cases explode in geometric proportions. Previously characterised as a self limiting disease, it appeared in more aggressive form during the epidemic since 2005. Vector borne disease such as Chikungunya and Dengue are the important infectious diseases in India. Chikungunya and Dengue vector control is possible by protecting the population from mosquito bite. However, at the national level, capacities to implement vector control programmes have been severely weakened, National vector control programmes often lack specialists in vector control and as a result, routine entomological activates such as surveillance or monitoring and evaluation of control activities are not conducted.

Extreme temperature is often lethal to the survival of disease causing pathogen but incremental change in temperature may exert varying effects. When temperature approaches to the limit of physiological tolerance for the pathogen, a small increase in temperature may be lethal to the pathogen. A small increase in temperature may result in increase in incubation, development and replication of the pathogen. Therefore increase of temperature increase their biting rates as well as vector population dynamics.

Symptoms

Chikungunya is featured by posture of bends upon the patients who are affected with severe joint pain frequently. The infection causes no symptoms at the early stage, especially in children. After recoveries from Chikungunya fever convalesce cane is prolonged and persistent. Infection appears to confer lasting immunity; Serological investigations are to be carried out to eliminate the possibility of other causes. The time between the bite of mosquito carrying Chikungunya virus and the start of symptoms ranges from 1 to 12 days.

Pathogenesis

Detailed information about pathogenesis of Chikungunya fever is not available. After the bite from an infected mosquito the virus multiplies in lymphoid and myeloid organs and subsequently induces cellular and humoral immunity which leads to manifestations of the disease.

Clinical Features

Fever

This disease occurs in all areas and in both sexes. Clinical features of Chikungunya fever are onset with high fever, headache and back pain, myalgia or intense pain in one or more joints, severe and crippling arthritis in hands and feet. Besides joint pain, other symptoms of the diseases are Fulminate hepatitis Mehingoencephalitis, Skin rash and Skin pigmentation. The posture of Chikungunya fever is bends up on the patients who are affected with a severe joint pain.

Figure 3.5: Swollen ankles and feet

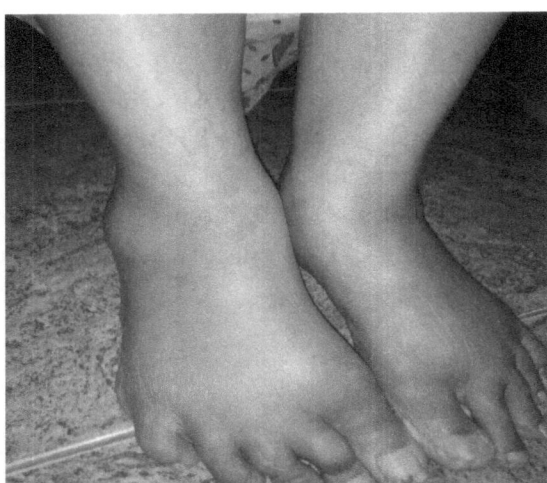

As per the guidelines from government, health authorities issued that epidemic suspect case of Chikungunya is one who presents with acute onset of high grade fever for less than 7 days duration associated with headache, arthralgias and myalgias, with or without rash. Probable case is defined as one coming from high vector density area or areas which confirm cases having clinical features of Chikungunya fever.

Rash

Chikungunya disease may present in two stages. At the initial stage severe eruptive polyrathritis followed by disabling peripheral rheumatism that can persist for months. Other dermatological features observed during outbreaks in southern India are nasal blotchy erythema, freckle like pigmentation over control facial area, flagellate.

Pigmentation on fare and extremities, lichenoid eruption and hyperpigmentatin in photo distributed are exilla and unior bilateral lymphedema in acral distribution. Multiple ecchynotic spots (in children) resiculobullous lesious (in infants) subungual hemorrhages photourticaria, acral urticaria and scaling with dyschromic patches have also been described.

The time between the bite of mosquito carrying Chikungunya virus and the start of symptoms ranges from 1 to 12 days without swelling or pain in the joints. It is very rare for the patients to relieve completely from various side effects immediately after recovery. Patients have joint pain for much longer period depending on their age.

Towards the end of 3rd to 5th day most patients are said to develop irritating rash commonly on the arms, back and shoulders and occasionally over the entire body. It usually lasts for 48 hours. Some studies show dermatological manifestations of pigmentary changes and brown-black pigmentations. Children may develop rash on the first day of the illness.

Arthritis

The joint pain is one of the important symptoms of Chikungunya fever. It may be severe and can never prevent sleep in the first few days of the illness. Patients develop articular symptoms and incapacitating joint pains lasting weeks to months. The involvement is polyarticular, more frequently in the lower limps and in small joints. (Mohan, 2006; Thiruvengadam Rt al, 1965; Kamath et al, 2006).

Swelling or pain in the joints is a major feature of Chikungunya fever. There can be mild haemorrhaging in children, joint pain can persist for many months or even years after the other symptoms have subsided. It is very rare for the patients to relieve completely from various side effects. After recovery patients have joint pain for much longer period depending on their age.

It is very rare for the patients to relieve completely from various side effects immediately after recovery. Patients have joint pain for much longer period depending on their age.

Other components of the musculoskeletal system may get involved presenting as tenosynovitis, bursitis, and soft tissue pain over arms, thighs and feet and occasionally tenderness over shin of tibia. Arthritis is usually severe enough to immobilise the patient. Most patients usually recover from arthritis within 2-3 weeks however, prolonged arthralgia testing beyond 4 months are seen in 12 – 13 percent and destructive arthropathy can occur in a few. In the absence of widespread availability of diagnostic test for Chikungunya, diagnosis is essentially clinical; epidemiology of diseases caused by Alfa viruses is highly specific and gives a clue to the diagnosis. It should be suspected in all patients with febrile polyarthritis with recent history of travel to areas with Chikungunya virus transmission.

The back, knees and ankles and feet become intensely painful. Although fever and skin-rash are short-lasting, the joint pains may recur or linger for a long time. Chik and Dengue viruses can coexist or co infection with Chikungunya and Dengue.

Hemorrhagic Manifestations

A classic case of Chikungunya fever is not to produce hemorrahagic manifestations. However, the outbreaks of Calcutta in 1963-64, in Thailand and Burma showed that adult patients and children developed these symptoms. This indicates that Chikungynya can cause heomorrahagic disease characterising bleeding. It was also observed that bleeding manifestations were less severe in Chikungunya patients when compared to Dengue.

Neurological Manifestations

The Chikungunya fever is responsible for severe morbidity during acute stage and causes systemic involvement including neurological complications. It has a long term impact on musculoskeletal system causing crippling arthritis.

Neurological Manifestations are not very common in Chikungunya. However some adults and children developed neurological complications which include febrile convulsions, altered level of consciousness, blindness due to retrobulbar neuritis and acute flaccid paralysis. (Ganesan et al, 2008).

Other Manifestations

Despite the high prevalence of Chikungunya infection, there are no studies on the socio economic profile in the spread of the disease or cost of morbidity experienced. Chikungunya fever emerged in many of the coastal states of India mainly due to water storing, migration, ecological reasons and immunity in the population. Hence they are more susceptible to the disease. Some studies stated that individual with poor background had serious consequence of Chikungunya fever. Much of the central government funds allotted to fight Chikungunya remain unused during the epidemic because of the absence of a proper plan.

General manifestations are like fatigability, weakness, loss of appetite, backache, body ache, restlessness, giddiness and hypotension, puffy face and edema feet. Imphadenopathy are usually present. This may be accompanied by pharyngitis gingivitis oral ulcerations.

Diagnosis

A clear case definition for Chikungunya has been developed by World Health Organisation (WHO) in three categories viz, suspected, probable and confirmed. Virus isolation, serological test and molecular technique of Polymerase Chain Reaction (PCR), are the three main laboratory tests used for diagnosing Chikungunya fever. The role of laboratory diagnosis is essential to differentiate the cases of Chikungunya into the three categories. Virus isolation, serological test and molecular technique of Polymerase Chain Reaction (PCR), are the three main laboratory tests used for diagnosing Chikungunya fever.

For serological diagnosis, serum obtained from 10-15 ml of blood is required. In the acute phase, serum must be collected immediately after the onset of illness and the convalescent phase serum 10-14 days later.

Virus isolation is the most definitive test. Between 2-5 ml of whole blood is collected during the first week of illness in commercial heparinised tube and transported on ice to the laboratory. Recently a reverse transcriptase RT-PCR technique for diagnosing Chikungunya virus has been developed using nested primary pairs amplifying specific components of three structural gene regions.

The other common viral illness similar to Chikungunya fever is infection by o'nyong-nyog virus. This infection can be differentiated on the basis of circulation of the o'nyong-nyong virus in the community at the time of clinical diagnosis and confirmation by the serological diagnosis. O'nyong-nyong virus is also different from Chikungunya virus as it is transmitted by anopheline mosquitoes. Sometimes, similar clinical presentation is made by Sindbis virus infection. The confirmatory diagnosis of Chikungunya fever from Dengue or o'nyong-nyong can be made by the laboratory investigation only.

The probable diagnosis of Chikungunya fever can be made on the basis of presence of the virus in community, a clinical trial of fever rashes and arthralgia. Confirmation of the illness is done by detection of the antigen or antibody to the agent in the blood sample of patient. Reverse transcriptase polymerase chain reaction (RT-PCR) is confirmatory for the identification of Chikungunya virus. IgM capture ELISA is the most sensitive serologic assay, and is necessary to distinguish the disease from Dengue. Although such precautions may not be necessary in the countries where Chikungunya virus is endemic, Chikungunya is the challenge to diagnosis because its symptoms are similar to other mosquito borne diseases like Dengue and Malaria. Hence accurate diagnosis is essential in order to minimise the spread of the disease.

New diseases like Chikungunya set confusion among health care providers and affected households. The confirmation of the disease by conducting tests is very rare because of the non-availability of testing centres locally. Hence the treatment is seldom based on testing but on symptomatic basis.

Treatment

There is no specific treatment for Chikungunya; Symptomatic treatment is recommended after excluding more serious conditions. Symptomatic or supportive treatment basically comprises rest and use of acetaminophen or paracetamol to relieve fever and ibuprofen, naproxen or other non-steroidal anti inflammatory agent (NSAID) to relieve the arthritic component. Joint pain may require analgesic and long-term anti-inflammatory therapy. Movement and mild exercise tend to improve morning stiffness and pain, but more exercise may exacerbate symptoms.

Chikungunya vs. Dengue

An Aegypti can maintain the virus in a human-mosquito – human cycle. Chikungunya and Dengue fever can occur together in the same patient. In Chikungunya, cases of shock or severe haemorrhage are not observed. The duration of fever is much shorter in the case of Chikungunya fever. In Chikungunya fever maevlopapular rash is more frequent than dengue fever.

All the clinical manifestation of Chikungunya fever resembles those of Dengue and other fever. Laboratory confirmation is critical to establish the infection of Chikungunya fever. It involves more cost and time. Hence symptomatic treatment is a common methodology for treatment.

The clinical illness of Chikungunya fever needs to be differentiated from Dengue and its variants. Rashes occur in both the disease but are more common in Chikungunya in which, decreases platelet count leads to the severe Haemorrhagic signs. Similarly, there is no retro orbital pain, a characteristic of Dengue; severe joint pain may or may not be associated with swellings is another characteristics of Chikungunya fever.

Chikungunya fever has to be distinguished from the Dengue fever which has the potential for much worse outcomes including death. Chikungunya and Dengue fever sometimes occur together in the same patient. All the clinical manifestation of Chikungunya fever resembles those of Dengue and some other fevers as well. The clinical illness of Chikungunya fever needs to be differentiated from dengue and its variants. Rashes occur in both the disease but are more common in Dengue. Decreases of platelet count leads to the severe haemorrhagic signs. Similarly, there is no retro orbital pain, a characteristic of Dengue in Chikungunya fever.

It is found that there is a progressive decrease in the cases of Malaria since 2005 in Tamil Nadu. But there is an increase in the case of either Dengue or Chikungunya. The government of Tamil Nadu evolved strategies and plan to tackle the breeding of vectors to prevent their spread. The Malaria causing anopheleses has been replaced by Aedes mosquitoes which cause Chikungunya or Dengue. In 2005 Tamil Nadu recovered nearly 40000 cases of Malaria, which came down to about 28000 in 2006, that year changed the monsoon disease dynamics by having maximum number of Chikungunya cases. The spread of Malaria, Dengue and Chikungunya in Chennai City is shown in Table 3.2.

Table 3.2: Spread of infectious disease in Chennai City

Year	Malaria	Dengue	Chikungunya
2009	483	326	440
2008	21046	640	71
2007	22389	707	45
2006	28219	477	64802
2005	39678	1150	-

Source: Chennai Corporation

Vector borne disease such as Chikungunya and Dengue are the important infectious diseases in India. Chikungunya and Dengue vector control is possible by protecting the population from mosquito bite. However, at the national level, capacities to implement vector control programmes have been severely weakened, National vector control programmes often lack specialists in vector control and as a result, routine entomological activates such as surveillance or monitoring and evaluation of control activities are not conducted.

References

Jhadhav M, Namboodripad M, Carmen R.H, Carey D.E, Mysers R.M, 1965, 'Chikungunya Disease in Infants and children in Vellore: A Report of Clinical Features of Virollogically Proved Cases', *Indian Journal of Medical Research*, 53, pp. 729-744.

Mohan A, 2006, 'Chikungunya Fever: Clinical Manifestations and Management', *Indian Journal of Medical Research*, 124, pp. 471-474.

Thiruvengadam K.V, Kalyanasundaram V, Rajagopal J, 1965, 'Clinical and Pathological Studies in Chikungunya Fever in Madras City', *Indian Journal of Medical Research*, 53, pp 729-744.

Kamat S, Das A.K, Parikh F.S, 2006, *Chikungunya*, JAPI, 54,pp 725-726.

Ganesan K, Diwan A, Shankar S.K, Desai S.B, Sainani G.S, Kartak S.M, 2008, 'Chikungunya Encephalomyeloradicultis: Report of 2 Cases with Neuroimaging and 1Case with Autopsy Findings', *AJNR American Journal of Neuroradiol.*

Powers AM, Logue CH, 2007, 'Changing Patterns of Chikungunya Virus: Re-emergence of a Zoonotic Arbovirus,' *Journal of Genetic Virology*, 88 pp.2363-2377.

.Lee HL, Vasan SS, Murtola TM, Field RW, Mavalankar DV, (et al.) 2008 Estimated Immediate Cost of Dengue and Chikungunya to Malaysia, *Unpublished observations*

Armien B, Suaya JA,Quiroz EQ, San BK, Bayard V, (et al), 2008, 'Clinical Characteristics and National Economics Cost of the 2005 Dengue Epidemic in Panama' *AM J Tropical Medicines and Hygiene*, 73, pp.364-371.

Mavalankar D, Shastri P, Bandyopadhyay T, Par mar J, Ramani K.V, 2008, 'Increased Mortality Rate Associated with Chikungunya Epidemic, Ahmadabad, India' *Emerging Infectious Disease*, 14(13)

Lum L.S, Suaya J.A, Lian H.T, San B.K, Sheppard D.S, 2008, 'Quality of Life of Dengue Patients' *American Journal of Tropical Medicine and Hygiene*, 78, pp.862-7.

Ross RW, 1956, 'The Newalla epidemic 111; The Virus: Isolation, Pathogenic properties and relationship to the epidemic', *Journal of Hygiene*, 54, pp.177-91.

Diallo M, Thonnon J, Traore Laminana M, Fonteille D, 1999, 'Vectors of Chikungunya Virus in Senegal: Current Data and Transmission Cycles', *AMJ Tropical Medicine Hygiene*, 60,pp. 281-6.

Mathew T, Tiruvengadam K.V, 1973, 'Further Studies on the Isolate of Chikungunya from the Indian Repatriates of Burma', *Indian Journal of Medical Research*, 61 (4), pp. 517-20.

Lam S.K, Chua K.B, Hooi P.S, 2001, 'Chikungunya Infection: Emerging Disease in Malasiya', *Southeast Asian Journal of Tropical Medicine Pus Health*, 32 pp.447-51.

Padbidri V.S, Gnaneswar T.T, 1979, 'Epidemiological Investigation of Chikungunya Epidemic at Barsi- Maharashtra State, India', *Journal of Hygienic Epidemiology Microbial Immunology*, 23(4), pp.445-51.

Ravi V, 2006, 'Reemergence of Chikungunya Virus in India,' *Indian Journal of Medical Microbial*, 24 (2) pp.83-4.

Parvi K, 1986, 'Disappearance of Chikungunya Virus from Indian and Southeast Asia', *Trans R Soc Tropical Med Hygiene*, 80, pp.491.

Singh K.V, Parvi K.M, 1967, 'Experimental Studies with Chikungunya Virus in Aedes aegypti and Aedes albopictus', *Acta Virol*, 11,pp. 517-26.

Mourya D.T, 1987, 'Absense of Transovarial Transmission of Chikungunya Virus in Aedes aegypti and Ae. Albopictus', *Indian Journal of Medical Research*, 85,pp. 593-5.

Kirshnamoorthy K, Nanda B, Subramanian S, 2008, Chikungunya Emergence inRural South India: Epidemiology- Ogy and Clinical Profile, *Indian Journal of Medical Research* (in press).

Brignton S.W, Porzesky O.W, Harpe A.L, 1982, 'Chikungunya Virus Infection: A Retrospective Study of 107 Cases,' *South African Medical Journal*, 63, PP. 313-5.

Pialoux G, Gauzere B.A, Jaureguiberry S, Strobel M, 2007, 'Chikungunya, an Epidemic Arbovirosis,' *Lancet infect Dis*, 7(5), pp. 319-27.

Kalantri S.P, Joshi R, Riley L.W, 2006, 'Chikungunya Epidemic an Indian Perspective', *National Medical Journal of India*, 19, pp. 315-22.

Gubler DJ, Meltzer M, 1999, 'Impact of Dengue / Dengue Hemorrhagic Fever on the Developing World,' *Adv virus Re*, 53, pp.35-70.

Zaidi A.K.M, Awasthi S, Desilva H.J, 2004, 'Burden of Infection Diseases in South Asia,' *Bangladesh Medical Journal*, 328, pp. 811-5.

Kalantri S.P, Joshi R, Riley L.W, 2006, 'Chikungunya Epidemic an Indian Perspective,' *National Medical Journal of India*,19, pp.315-22.

Adhikari S.R, Maskay N.M, 2003, 'The Economic Burden of Kalazan in Household of the Danusna and Mahottari Districts of Nepal,' *Acta Trop*, 88 pp.1-2.

WHO- SEARO, 2007, Communicable Diseases, *Newsletter,* 4(3)pp.1-5.

Pialoux G, Gauzere B.A, Jaureguiberry S, Strobel M, 2007, 'Chikungunya, an Epidemic Aarbovirosis,' *Lancet infects Dis,* 7 (5), pp. 319-27.

Krishna M.R, Reddy M.K and Reddy S.R, 2006, Chikungunya Outbreaks in Andrapradesh, *South India current Science,* 91(5) pp.570-571.

Robinson M.C, 1955, 'An Epidemic of Virus Disease in Southern Province, Tanganjika Territory, in 1952-53, Clinical Features' *Trans R Soc Trop Med Hyg,* 49 pp.28-32.

Halstead S.B, Scanlon J.E, Umpaivit Pand Udomsakdi S, 1969, 'Dengue and Chikungunya Virus in Man in Thailand, 1962-64. IV, Epidemiologic Area,' *American Journal of Tropical Medicine and Hygiene,* 18(6) PP. 997-1021.

World Health Organization - South- East Asia Regional Office, 2008, 'Chikungunya in South East Asia update'.

World Health Organization, 2007, 'Outbreak and Spread of Chikungunya,' Weakly Epidemiological Records, 82 (47) pp.409-415.

Pialoux G, Gauzere B.A, Jaurequiberry S and Stobel M, 2007, 'Review: Chikungunya an Epidemic Arbovirosis, *Lancet infect Dis,* 7, pp. 319-27.

Yergollcar P, Tandale B, Arankalle V, (et al), 2006, 'Chikungunya outbreaks caused by African genotype, India', *Emerge in fact Dis,* 12, pp. 1580-83.

Mohan A, 2006, Editorial- Chikungunya Fever,Clinical Manifestation and Management, *Indian Journal of medical Research,* 124:471-474.

Swaroop A, Jain A, Kumar M, Parihar N, and Jain S, 2007, Review Article, 'Chikungunya Fever', *Indian Academy of clinical medicine,* 8(2) pp.164-68.

Kennedy A.C, Fleming J, and Solomon L, 1980, 'Chikungunya Viral Arthropathy: A Chemical Description,' *J Rheumatol,* 7(2) pp. 231-36.

Simon F, Parole P, Granddame M, (et al.), 2007, 'Chikungunya Infection: An Emerging Rheumatism among Travelers Returned from Indian Ocean Islands, Report of 47 Cases', *Medicine* (Baltimore), 86(3) pp. 123-37.

Mahendradas P, Ranganna S, Shetty R, (et al.), 2008, Ocular Manifestations Associated with Chikungunya', *Ophthalmology,* 115(2) pp. 287-291.

Wadia R.S, 2007, Presidential Oration: A Neurotropic Virus (Chikungunya) and a Neurotropic Amino acid (homocysteine)', *Ann India head neurol,* 10, pp. 198-213.

Gerardin P, Baraurer, Michault A,(et al),2006, 'Multi- disciplinary Prospective Study of Mother-to-Child Transmission of Chikungunya

Virus Infections on the Island of La Reunion,' *PLOS Medicine,* Vol.5, No 3 eto doi: 10.1371/ Tournal.pmed.0050060.

Ramful D, Carbonnier M, Pasquet,(et. al), 2007, 'Mother-to-child Transmission of Chikungunya Virus Infections', *Prediator Infect Dis Journal,* 26 (9), pp. 811-15.

Lenglet Y, Barau G. Robillard P.Y, (et al.), 2006, 'Chikungunya Infection in Pregnancy: Evidence for Intrauterine Infection in Pregnant Women and Vertical Transmission in Parturient: Survey of the Reunion Island Outbreak,' *J Gynecol Obstet Biol Ne prods* (Paris), 35(A) pp. 578-83.

Khursed P, 1986, Disappearance of Chikungunya Virus from India and South East Asia,' *Trans Royal Soc Trop Med Hyg,* 80, P. 491.

Park K. Parks, 2005, *Text book of Preventive and Social Medicine,* in Bhanot B.D, editor. 18th ed. Jabalpur.

Dandawate C.N, Thiruvengadam K.V, Kalyansundram V, Rajagopal J, Rao TR, 1965, 'Serological Survey in Madras City with Special reference to Chikungunya', *Indian med res,* 53, pp.707-14.

Josseran,L,.C.Paquet, A.zehgnoun,N.Caillere,A. Le Terte, J.solet, and M.Ledrans, 2006 'Chikungunya Disease Outbreak, Reunion Island, Emerging infections Diseases.12:1994.

Robinson Marion, 1955, 'An Epidemic of Virus Diseases in Southern Provinoe, Tanganyika Territory, in 1952-53; I, Clinical Features,' *Trans Royal society Trop med Hyg,* 49:28-32.

Parik, 1986, 'Disappearance of Chikungunya Virus from India and Southern Asia,' *Trans R Soc Trop med Hyg*; 80, P.491.

Yergolkar PN,Tandale BV,Arankalle V.A,(et al.), 2006, 'Chikungunya Outbreaks Caused by African Genotype, India,' *Emerge infect Dis,* 12, pp.1580-3.

Neogi D.K, Bhatta Charya N, Mukherjee K.K, (et al),2006, 'Sero Survey of Chikungunya Antibody in Calcutta Metropolis,' *J Commun Dis,* 1995,37, pp.19-22.

Schuffenecker I, Iteman I, Michault A, Murris, Frangeul L, Vaney MC,2006, (et. al), 'Genome Microevolution of Chikungunya Viruses Causing the Indian Ocean outbreak, *PLOS Med,* 3, P.263.

Banerjee K, Mourya D.T, Malunjkar, 1988, 'As Susceptibility and Transmissibility of Different Geographical Strains of Aedes aegypti Mosquitoes to Chikungunya Virus India', *Journal of Medical Research*, 87, pp.134-8.

Singh N, Shukla M.M, Mishra A.K, Singh M. P, Pailwal J.C, Dash A. P, 2006, 'Malaria Control Using Indoor Residual Sprajing and Carnivorous Fish: A Case study in Betel, Central India', *Tropical Medicine Internal Health,* 11, pp.1512-2.

Gibbons R.V, Vaughn D.W, 2002, 'Dengue: An Escalating Problem', *Bangladesh Medical Journal*, 324, pp. 1563-6.

Wilder Smith A, Schwartz E, 2005, 'Dengue in Travelers', *N English Journal of Medicine*, 353, pp. 924-32.

Zytoon E.M, El-Belbasi H.I, Matsumura T,1993 'Mechanism of Increased Dissemination of Chikungunya Virus in Aedes albopictus Mosquitoes Concurrently Ingesting Microfilariae of Dirofilaria Immitis' *American Journal of Tropical Medicine and Hygiene*, 49, pp. 201-7.

Mishra B, Ratho R.K, 2006, 'Chikungunya Reemergence: Possible Mechanism,' *Lancet,* 368, P. 918.

Higgs S, 2006, 'The 2005-2006 Chikungunya Epidemic in the India Ocean' *Vector Borne Zoonatic Dis*, 6, pp. 115-16.

Mourya D.T,Mishra A.C, 2006, 'Chikungunya Fever,' *Lancet,* 368, pp. 186-7.

Brighton S.W, 1981, 'Chikungunya Virus Infections,' *South African Medical Journal*, 59, P.552.

Thaikruea L, Charearnsook O, Reanphum Karnkit S, Dissomboon P, Phonjan R, Ratchbud S, (et al) 1997, 'Chikungunya in Thailand A Reemerging Disease,' *South East Asian Journal of Tropical Medicine and Public Health*, 28, pp. 359-64.

Kumarasamy V, Pathapa S, Zuridah H, Chem Y.K, Norizah I, Chua K.B, 2006, 'Reemergence of Chikungunya Virus in Malaysia,' *Medical Journal of Malaysia*, 61, pp.221-5.

Fradin M.S,Day J.F, 2002, 'Comparative Efficacy of Insect: Repellent Against Mosquito Bites,' *N English Journal of Medicine*, 347, pp.13-18.

Benenson A. S, 1995, 'Control of Communicable Diseases in Man', 16 Ed., USA, *American Public Health Association*.

Campos L E, San Juan A, Cenabre L.C, Alrnagro E.E, 1969, 'Isolation of Chikungunya Virus in the Philippines,' *Acta Med Philipp,* 552(4), pp.152-155.

Saxena S.K. Singh M, Mishra N, Lakshmi V, 2006, 'Resurgence of Chikungunya Virus in India: An Emerging Threat', *Euro surveill,* 11:E060810.2.

Krishna M.R, Reddy M.K, Reddy S.R, 2006, 'Chikungunya Outbreaks in Andhra Pradesh, South India,' *Current Science,* 91(5), pp.570-571.

'Outbreak and Spread of Chikungunya, 2007, *'Weekly Epidemiological Record,* 82 (47) pp. 409-415.

Mohan A, 2006, 'Chikungunya fever; Clinical Manifestations and Management,' *India Journal of Medical Research,* 124(5) pp.471-4.

Swaroop Jain A, Kumhar M, Parihar N, Jain S, 2007, 'Chikungunya Fever' *Journal of Indian Academy of Clinical Medicine,* 8(2), pp.164-68.

Kennedy A.C, Fleming J, Solomon L, 1980, 'Chikungunya Virus Arthropathy: A Clinical Description,' *Journal of Rheumatology,* Mar-Apr; 7(2), pp. 231-6.

Mahendradas P, Ranganna S.K, Shetty R, Balu R, Narayana K.M, Babu R B, Shetty B.K,2008, 'Ocular Manifestations Associated with Chikungunya', *Ophthalmology Fed;* 115(2), pp.287-9.

Pialoux G, Gauzere B. A, Jaureguiberrys, Straubel M, 2007, 'Chikungunya An Epidemic Arbovirosis, *Lancet Infect Dis,* Issues (5) No, pp.319-27.

Mohan A, 2006, 'Chikungunya Fever: Clinical Manifestation and Management,' *India J med Res,* No.124.

Ravi V, 2006, 'Re- emergence of Chikungunya Virus in India,' *J med Microbial,* Vol; 24, No, 83-4.

Mourya D.T, Mishra A. C, 2006, 'Chikungunya Fever', *Lancet,* Vol.368, No 187-7.

Bodemman P, Genton B, 2006, 'Chikungunya: An Epidemic in Real Time' *Lancet,* No, 368.

Enserink M, 2006, 'Massive Outbreak Draws Fresh Attention to Little Known Virus', *'Science,* Vol.311, No, 1085.

Gersoviz, Mark, 2000, 'A Preface to the Economic Analysis of Disease Transmission', *Australian Economic Papers,* Vol.39, issue, 1.

Gerpvotz, Mark,Hammer, Jeffrey S, 2004, 'The Economical Control of infectious Diseases,' *Economic Journal,* Vol.114, Issue, 492.

Climate Change, Chikungunya And Vector Management

The influence of climate change in infectious diseases has been a serious topic of discussion. There are sufficient literature points out the relationship between warmer temperature and change in rainfall pattern and transmission of certain vectors critical to the spread of infectious diseases. The poor socio-economic conditions of people in tropical countries work in support of the infliction of infectious diseases.

The short variations in climate conditions and extreme weather events can increase mortality, physical injury, mental health and other health outcomes. Changes in climate can affect human health through infectious disease transmission. Infectious agents receive the necessary nutrients from higher organism. Most such infections are benign. Only a few infections adversely affect the host's "biology" that is termed as infectious diseases.

The effect of climate change on infectious diseases is determined by transmission cycle. The transmission cycle of each pathogen is transmitted by a cycle which requires a vector or non-human host that are susceptible to external environmental influence. The infectious diseases are caused at the one side by the pathogen and the other side the human.

Most of the environmentally influencing factors for the spread of these diseases are temperature, precipitation and humidity. The following chart 4.1.explains the four main types of transmission cycle for infectious disease.

Figure 4.1: Transmission cycle of infectious diseases Anthroponoses

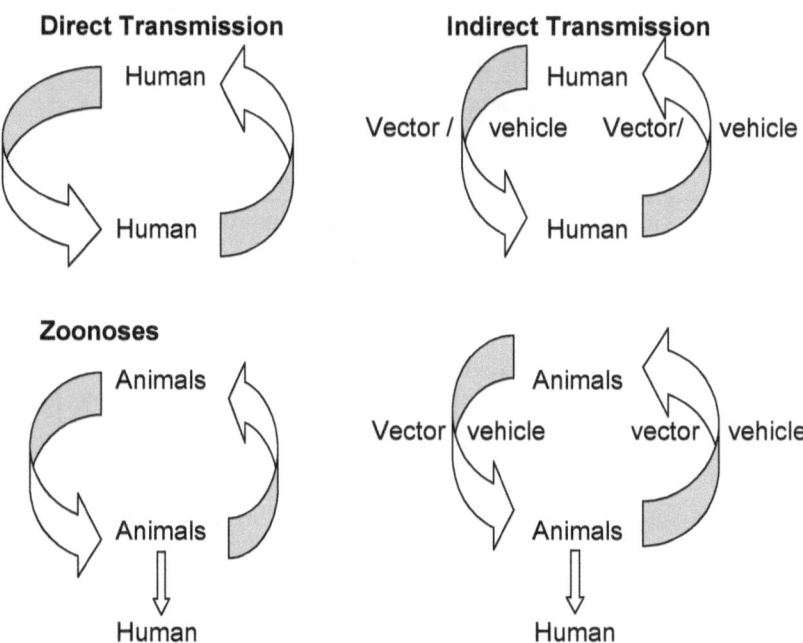

Climate change is a possibility and if the temperature increases at different levels, it will have different impact on human health. The reports of Intergovernmental Panel on Climate Change (IPCC) presented different levels of temperature increase subjected to the varied levels in the emission of greenhouse gases. The impact on increasing temperature on human health is described in the 5th report of the IPCC. The effect of temperature increase on health is shown in chart 4.1.

Climate change is a definite phenomenon that creates extreme weather pattern and global warming. These extreme weather patterns and global warming have a direct negative impact on infectious diseases especially vector-borne infectious diseases. This resurgence and redistribution of the mosquito puts an extra pressure on the public health system especially, the public health infrastructure of a developing country.

Chart 4.2: Effects of temperature increase on health

Temperature	Human health
1°C	At least 30,000 people each year die from climate related disease (Predominantly Diarrhea, Malaria, and malnutrition)
2° C	40-60 million more people exposed to Malaria in Africa
3°C	1-3 million more people die from malnutrition (if forbilisation weak)
4° C	Up to 80 million more people exposed to malaria in Africa
5° C	further disease increase and substantial burdens on health care services

Sources: Stern, 2007: IPCC 2007.

Climate is the average weather, described in terms of the mean and other statistical quantities that measure the variability over a period of time and possibly over a certain geographical region (Chan et al 19999). According to Epstein (2001) climate is key determinant, and climate constrains the range of infectious diseases, while weather affects the timing and intensity of outbreaks. The WHO has reported that since 1975 over 30 new diseases have appeared. In addition there has been a resurgence of old diseases such as Malaria, Chikungunya and Cholera. Of course, a resurgence and redistribution of infectious diseases is partly due to the deterioration of the public health delivery system. Human and mosquitoes contact reflects changing ecological and climate conditions as well as social changes (Epstein, 2001).

Vector born diseases would pose the greatest threat to human being transmitted by Aedes aegypti mosquitoes such as Chikungunya, Dengue and Yellow fever. The limiting factor in the spread of these epidemics was the onset of very cold and very hot weather. Aedes aegypti mosquitoes are killed rapidly at freezing temperature. The development of mosquito larvae is faster in moderate warm climate; therefore with global warming, the mosquitoes will spread in larger areas and most of the months in a year. In addition to transmission of the viruses in larger geographic area, the incubation period of dengue and Chikungunya viruses are dependent on temperature. The warmer the ambient temperature, shorter is the incubation period. From the time the mosquito imbibes the infective blood, the mosquito is able to transmit the disease only by bite.

The viruses of Chikungunya, Yellow Fever and Dengue would have a shorter extrinsic incubation period and thus would cycle more rapidly in the mosquito. A more rapid cycle would increase the speed of epidemic spread. With global climate change, the vector will become more prevalent and extend its range even further in the North Pole compounding the risk of transmission. There is a perception that global climate change will be associated with areas of drought thus Aedes aegypti will not have sufficient water in which to breed. However, it is paradoxical that this mosquito thrives both in wet and dry climate. The mosquito is domestic and breeds in water storage, flower pots etc. Therefore, the infectious diseases are the problem of the poor tropical countries at present but this will spread to the cold countries when their temperatures hit up.

The future burden of diseases by 2030 will be 10 percent more diarrhoeal diseases than there would have been with no climate change. These diseases will affect primarily the young children, if global temperature increases by 2 to 3°C. As expected, it is estimated that the population at risk for Malaria will increase by 3 to 5 percent which means that millions of additional people would probably become infectious with Malaria each year.

Health Care Delivery

A framework is necessary for the public health sector to forecast the risks of epidemics in different demographic and geographic regions. Malaria is an interesting vector-borne disease, brings up the issue of the preparedness of and their developing countries capabilities to handle the epidemic stemming from climate change. Though Malaria and Dengue have a clear medical history, new diseases like Chikungunya generate doubts among the medical practitioners in the beginning. The range and transmission of mosquitoes has been affected by global warming mostly in developing countries. If the public health infrastructure does not anticipate the effects of climate change on infectious diseases, millions of people could die and millions of workdays will be lost. Climate change is a global issue and must be dealt with things before they go wrong. There are clear-cut evidences showing changes in environment leading to the emergence of infectious diseases by changes in the pathway of effect. Chart 4.2 shows examples of environmental changes and possible effects on infectious diseases.

The geography and history of infectious diseases shows that they are prevalent in places where the weather is hot and wet and where the people are poor (WHO, 2005). Climate determines the potential of flourishing many infectious diseases while health care influences the actual incidence of disease. One would therefore expect that in a scenario of economic growth, infectious diseases would fall as health care improves (Medlin et al., 2006). Likewise, in a scenario of global warming, one would expect to see infectious diseases spread into new regions and perhaps intensify (McMichael at al., 2001). In a scenario with both growth and warming, it is unclear what to expect, but projections of future disease incidence should take both into account. Previous studies suffer from the oversimplification of equating 'development' with 'economic growth'.

This limitation by driving the evolution of a few of the statistically significant underlying determinants of adaptive capacity into the future along economic growth scenarios and tracking the resulting vulnerability of two diseases – Malaria and Diarrhoea.

Chart 4.3: Environmental changes and infectious diseases

Environmental	Diseases	Changes pathway effect
Dams, canals, irrigation	Schistosomiasits Malaria Helminthiasies River blindness	Snail host habitat, human contact Breeding sites for mosquitoes Larval contact due to moist soil Blackfly breeding, disease
Agricultural intensification	Malaria Venezuelan haemorraghic fever	Crop insecticides, vector resistance Rodent abundance, contact
Urbanisation, urban crowding	Cholera Dengue	Sanitation, hygiene; Water contamination Water –collecting trash
Deforestation and new habitation	Cutaneous leishmaniasis Malaria	Aedes Aegypti mosquito breeding sites Proximity, sand fly vectors Breeding sites and vectors, immigration of susceptible people Contact, breeding of vectors Contact with sand fly vectors
	Oropouche Visceral leishmaniasis	Tick hosts, outdoor exposure Toxic algal blooms Pools for mosquito breeding
Reforestation Ocean warming Elevated precipitation	Lyme disease Red tide Rift valley fever Hantavirus pulmonary syndrome	Rodent food, habitat, abundance

Source: Wilson, Ecosystem Change and Public Health: A Global Perspective, 2001.

Adaptive Capacity

Adaptation is one of the methodologies evolved to meet the effects of possible global warming and climate change. The term 'adaptive capacity' was coined by Smith et al (2001) in the context of impacts of climate change. Impacts follow from the combination of (i) being exposed to a particular manifestation of climate change (e.g., an increase in the number of Malaria-carrying mosquitoes) and (ii) being vulnerable to that.

Adaptive capacity is the ability of a system to adapt to or cope with (climate) change, and is therefore a reflection of the potential to diminish vulnerability. Because neither adaptive capacity nor vulnerability is rigorously defined, we use adaptive capacity loosely as the inverse of vulnerability. The notion of adaptive capacity has proved useful in the study of the impacts of climate change. Essentially, adaptive capacity measures the ability of a society to respond, either to make the best of new opportunities opened by climate change, or to minimise the negative consequences. Adaptive capacity for climate change is similar to adaptive capacity for any change.

Risk of Spread to Distant Area

As the Aedes can fly only a few hundred meters, flying mosquitoes are unlikely to spread the disease across a large geographical area. More than the mosquito, the mobility of people influenced by the globalisation of trade and travel is largely responsible for the wide distribution of the virus.

Re-emergence of Chikungunya Fever and Climate

The emergence of Chikungunya disease in the coastal States of India is a fine case of the re-emergence of an infectious disease after a long gap probably due to more number of hot years in the last decade of the 20th century and in the initial years of the new millennium. The Chikungunya virus was first identified in Calcutta in 1963, subsequently in Vellore and Chennai of Tamil Nadu. After that the virus disappeared in the Indian subcontinent for more than 20 years. However this infectious disease re-emerged in several parts of South India, but it occurs in different parts of India thereafter. The chronology of the spread of the Chikungunya fever is shown in chart 4.4.

The Chikungunya fever is a dreaded disease even though the disease is treated as non-fatal. The incubation period of the disease is 2 to 4 days. The symptoms are severe in children than adults; its complications are acute among pregnant women and aged.

Infected patients manifest sudden onset of fever, chills, severe arthralgia and headache. Patients also have maculopapular rash mostly in trunk. Migratory polyrathritis (commonly swelling and reddening) occurs in 70 percent cases and mainly affected the small joints. They may also manifest photophobia, anorexia, nausea, conjunctival infection and abdominal pain.

The acute illness usually last for 5 to 7 days. Chikungunya has not been reported causing severe haemorrhagic manifestation or death. Older patients usually continue to suffer recurrent joint pain effusion for several years. The economic burden of the disease is more after the recovery from fever and it takes long time for the patients to regain their original health status.

Chart 4.4: Chronology of Chikungunya outbreak in India

Year	Locality	Important Characteristics	Reference
1963	Calcutta	*Cases in Lakhs *37 percent naemmorrhage manifestation *Approx 200 deaths	KMR Bulletin May 1980
1964	Madras	*Cases in Lakhs *5.8 percent haemmorrhyage manifestation	Sarkar al IJMR 1964 (52), 651-660
1973	Maharashtra	*Small outbreak *No haemmorrhage manifestation	
2005	Andhra Pradesh Maharashtra Karnataka	*6421 cases *No haemmorrhage manifestation *34725 cases *No haemmorrhage manifestation *18529 cases	Investigation reports, NICD, Delhi.

Source: Ministry of Labour, Government of India.

The linking of the most important climate factor namely temperature with infectious diseases shows both direct and indirect relationship through ecological processes. A casual relationship between climate change and patterns of infectious diseases is cited by taking the re-emergence of Chikungunya fever. A comparative analysis of mosquito borne diseases shows the association of vector habits, disease patterns and climatic factors. The linkage between climate change and the spread of Chikungunya is useful for managing the infectious diseases due to changes in the temperatures. Mitigation and adaptation policies related to climate change influence the intensity of Chikungunya fever. The capacity of developed countries in health delivery system and environment management helped prevention of infectious diseases while these are the limitations in the case of developing countries.

Socio Economic Impact

Though Chikungunya is not a killer disease, high morbidity and prolonged polyarthritis and chronic illness cause severe socio-economic impact in the affected States. Hospital records suggest that children and elderly were the most severely affected group. Chikungunya fever occurs in all ages and both sexes. It is not considered as a fatal disease; hence adequate attention was not paid in the initial period leading to medical emergency. Public intervention measures such as distribution of mosquito nets, application of insecticide, sites sources reduction by fish production, constant monitoring and supervision, weekly reporting and surveillance system for fever and commitment from various government departments are indispensable during medical emergency of the outbreak of the epidemic. Since no effective vaccine or drugs available for treatment, prevention is the best available option to control the disease. Prevention is possible by early identification of outbreaks, vector control and continuous surveillance. Vector control is the most economical and the only way to prevent and control the outbreak of Chikungunya. In order to make prevention successful, guidelines need to be prepared for proper surveillance, clinical case management, and control and prevention of Chikungunya fever.

The most significant impact of Chikungunya fever affected households is the economic impact and distress caused by the disease. The disease worsens economic position of the people due to the health care cost, productivity loss and unemployment. The disease was at its peak during monsoon and winter month's when rural people are busy with agricultural activities. These months decide the earning levels of the rural people. Chikungunya stuck in these months rendering a majority of the rural populace incapacitated for a varying period of nearly 2 to 7 months.

Chikungunya equally affects landowner as well as the tillers. The spread of Chikungunya fever has serious effects on the labour scenario of the affected region. Loss of livelihood is comparatively more serious for the labourers as compared to the farmers because the labourers have practically no savings and usually live in a situation of hand to mouth existence. Many families, which usually do not migrate, are forced to migrate in search of employment to overcome the revenue loss during the sick period. Besides the impact on employment and income generation, Chikungunya fever causes marked loss in energy levels of people infected causing loss of productivity for a long period. In addition to the wage loss and productivity loss, many households were subjected to exploitation by the clinics and medical centres after assessing their panic situation. Private Doctors take advantage of the ignorance of the people. Disbelieves and superstitions also force the rural people into seasonal migration.

Government hospitals could not accommodate more patients hence majority of the poor households had to depend on private health care providers for curing the disease since the disease is new. Psychosis is common among the affected households. The private health providers successfully exploited the situation by conducting many unwarranted tests and advocating unnecessary medicines. The dependence of poor households on private hospitals increased the economic burden of the health care seeking households. Interviews with the affected households revealed that they prefer private medical care because they received poor health care delivery from government hospitals.

Nevertheless over reliance on private health care providers with inadequate infrastructural facilities is a common feature in rural areas. The high cost of private health care was not because of the income status of the households but severity of the disease compelled people to seek private medical care. The health care system needs a disaster management confront the challenge posed by sudden outbreak of the disease. Since the disease emerges for the first time in India, the outbreak was without any treatment history challenged the health care system.

Loss of livelihood opportunities of the affected households in the Kharrif and early Rabbi Season caused loss of food security and consequent indebtedness. Evaporation of credit access and lack of income earning opportunities are some of the important economic implications of Chikungunya fever. Though social and economic impact of Chikungunya fever is self limiting, high rate of morbidity results in heavy social and economic cost. The high socio-economic health burden of Chikungunya fever is mainly attributed to the higher disease burden in the areas of outbreak. Chikungunya is a vector borne-disease which shattered the livelihood of hundreds of thousands of people in 15 States between 2005 and 2008. It disproportionately affects the health of poor and marginalised populations. It serves as one of the serious health impediment to development. Climate changes in the form of increased climate variability, flood and stagnation of rain water cause the spread of communicable diseases mostly by mosquitoes and rodents.

The individuals affected with Chikungunya remain incapacitated at least for a week losing their occupation and income. The loss of income due to illness is used to calculate for those in the working age class. The household cost of illness is measured in terms of catastrophic out-of-packet health care expenditure, loss of productivity and wage loss. Chikungunya is a neglected tropical disease as there is little evidence about social, medical and economic implications as well as their impact. Even though the disease is rarely life-threatening, the widespread occurrence of the disease causes substantial morbidity and economic loss to the households.

The widespread episodes of Chikungunya fever impose huge economic burden on the households due to absenteeism and low productivity among workers. Poor households incur relatively large amount on treatment and transportation. In areas with limited access to medical facilities, households spend more on transportation and private medical care.

Chikungunya fever re-emerged for the first time in Andhra Pradesh subsequently with a series of outbreaks in most of the Coastal States of the rest of the country. As per the data from the National Vector Borne Disease Control Programme (NVBDCP) there were 104 million suspected and 1985 confirmed Chikungunya cases in 2006 to 2008 from 15 States and Union territories. The health system of the country was put into an important test, faced challenges in ensuring timely and rapid availability of standardised drugs, vaccines and diagnostic measures.

Since the disease emerged for the first time in the recent years, the health system had to confront more challenges in prevention and management of the outbreak. Measuring the loss of productivity is in terms of time and consequent loss of income. There is considerable loss of productive time even after the recovery from the fever. The loss of working time is acute during the phase of the illness and it continues even after the fever subsided.

The loss of work time after the recovery from fever is less than a full working day but in terms of loss of some hours.

The economic cost of Chikungunya fever is relatively high because of severe joint pain for long periods making it impossible for the patient to pursue their activities perfectly. The disease also caused loss to the national exchequer because of its impact on international tourism and trade. International travel and trade affected hoping that Chikungunya fever transmits in new areas.

Though productivity loss and wage loss are the important impacts of Chikungunya fever, household with multiple members affected with Chikungunya fever at a time is similar to a kind of trauma. The economic impact of the Chikungunya fever at the household level is very high due to multiple infected persons and the non- affected members taking the role of caretakers. Severe economic impact would be overpowering the poor households because of their inability to meet out the health cost on the one hand and earn for their livelihood on the other. Household economic cost of Chikungunya fever constitutes by out-of-packet health care expenditure and loss of productivity.

The widespread occurrence of the disease caused substantial morbidity and economic loss. Tamil Nadu, a South East coastal State of India has been witnessing the occurrence of the disease in different districts in different years since 2006. The disease emerged for the first time without a history of rapid outbreak made the health system to confront with more challenges in prevention and management of the outbreak.

The unavailability of prompt health care imposed a heavy economic burden both on the health system and on the households due to delay in treatment or management or mismanagement of treatment processes. The economic burden of Chikungunya fever varied from State-to-State depending upon the physical and financial infrastructural access to health care. It is reported by Medical authorities of Chikungunya affected states that the economic burden of the fever is even higher than that of some of the chronic non-communicable diseases, especially in the short-run.

A large proportion of the sick persons either consulted private health care professionals or sought alternative medical care and relatively less number consulted public health officials.

Initially hospitals were ill equipped to handle the burden of the epidemic. Many private hospitals thrived and arranged make-shift hospitals to accommodate sudden inflow of patients. The socio economic impact of the disease includes dropping of school attendance, sharp decline of productivity and severe stoppage of agricultural activities. Victims of Chikungunya fever lost their wages sold household assets and many of them were forced to borrow at high interest rates.

Agriculture is the worst affected sector due to the Chikunguniya fever because the disease occurs during the monsoon season when agricultural activities are at its peak. The mass spread of the fever in many localities made cultivations to get either delayed or postponed. All those infected by Chikunguniya fever were incapable of performing physical work in farms. This led to the stoppage of agricultural activities in many places. Labour shortage was recorded more than 40 percent in most of the Chikunguniya affected villages. Rubber plantations in Kanyakumari District of Tamil Nadu and Kottayam District of Kerala faced severe shortage of labourers when Chikunguniya fever was at its peak. Able but inefficient labourers demanded very high wages that made even cultivable lands to remain fallow.

The infection of Chikunguniya fever made the life of poor people very difficult. The small and marginal farmers in villages cultivate cereals for household consumption. The delay in sowing and failure to till the land forced them to purchase cereals from market. This made severe burden on their already poor economic conditions and caught them in the clutches of poverty-trap. In general, this had a resultant effect on the cash position and asset reserves of even the large farmers. The personal income of small and marginal farmers declined sharply and rural indebtedness penetrated into different sections of the society. A disastrous decline in the income of farming community effected reduction in the income of landless agricultural labourers, rural artisans, informal workers, petty traders and small shop owners. The socio-economic impact of Chikungunya fever is less known but it is severe in the form of school attendance drop, decline in productivity, and huge loss in the agriculture sector where farmers could not attend to their crops.

Chikungunya fever did not spare even the landlords due to the adverse effects of labour scarcity in these areas. However, the livelihood opportunities of the labourers were drastically affected. Many farmers kept their land fallow rather than tilled due to labour shortage. Theoretically this is an opportunity for the landless labourers to earn higher income but many of them were incapacitated to perform due to the infection of Chikungunya fever. The loss of livelihood of the labourers was more serious than the farmers because the former had practically no savings, usually lead a life of hand-to-mouth existence. The loss of revenue and need for credit forced farmers to sell their assets at low prices. Many sold cattle and portion of their land which would have physical and psychological implications for the farmers.

Chikungunya fever gave windfall gains for private doctors when the disease was rampant in rural areas. The disease has no vaccine or drugs therefore the medical cost of the disease is very less. However, due to the anxiety and suspicion of the disease, the victims were ready to take treatment in luxury hospitals. The economic burden of the disease is very high at the household level if direct and indirect costs of the illness are taken into account.

The economic burden of the disease is very high but it can be prevented. Multifaceted approach is necessary for preventing the disease both at the household and municipal level. The important but easy methods of prevention include:

Vector Management

Functioning of disease surveillance systems and effective environment health services are crucial in protecting public health in responding to the outbreak of a disease like Chikungunya. Integrated vector management is a process for managing vector populations in such a way as to reduce or interrupt transmission of disease. It consists of vector surveillance and vector control through better knowledge on the characteristics of vector biology, disease transmission, morbidity as well as a range of interventions and collaboration between all related parties. To prevent infecting others in the household or in the community, a patient of Chikungunya should strictly avoid coming in contact with an Aedes mosquito during the viremic phase, which is usually the first 4 days of illness. As the Aedes mosquito bites during dawn to-dusk daytime, sleeping in bed with a drug-impregnated net can interrupt the transmission of the disease. Vector control is not an easy task. But use of insecticide spraying is not always successful and effective. The aversive expenditure on vector prevention includes cost of mosquito nets, repellent, coils, spray, cream and other preventive measures. Preparedness measures can greatly increase the ability to control communicable disease such as Chikungunya fever.

The socio-economic factors and public health inadequacies facilitated the rapid spread of this infection. As it is a re-emerging disease, it has not received sufficient coverage, in the medical arena. The outbreak of

Chikungunya fever is seen as a political issue in the country without a proper disease management programme. Such an outbreak in every country would end-up by devising a proper rational policy on its prevention and control. New disease like Chikungunya set confusion among both health care providers and affected households.

REFERENCES

Andreano and Helminiak, 1988, 'Economic, Health and Tropical Disease; A Review in Economics', *Health and Tropical Disease*, University of Philippines School of Economics

Barron R, Sala-I-Martin X, 1995, *Economic Growth*, McGraw-Hill, New York.

Berndt, Ernst R, 2007, 'Advance Market Commitments for Vaccines against Neglected Diseases: Estimating Cost and Effectiveness', *Health Economics*, Vol, 16.Issues, 5.

Bhargava A, Jamison D, Lau L, Murray C, 2001, 'Modeling the Effects of Health on Economic Growth,' *Journal of Health Economics*, 20, pp.423-440.

Bloom DE, Canning D, 2006, 'Epidemics and Economics, Program on the Global Demography of Aging' *Working Paper No.9,* Harvard initiative for Global Health.

Bloom DE, Canning D, Seville J, 2004, 'The Effect of Health on Economic Growth: A Production Function Approach,' *World Development*, 32, pp.1-13.

Bodenmann P, Genton B, 2006, 'Chikungunya, An Epidemic in Real Time', *Lancet,* 368, P.258.

Brighton S.W, Prozesky O.W, de la Harpe A.L, 1983, 'Chikungunya Virus Infection A retrospective Study of 107 Cases,' *South African Medical Journal,* 63, pp.313-15.

Centre for Science and Environment, 2010, *Down to Earth,* 41, February pp.16 -28.

Cummings D.A, Irizarry R.A, Huang N.E, Endy T.P, Nisalak A, et al, 2004, 'Travelling Waves in the Occurrence of Dengue Hemorrhagic Fever in Thailand', *Nature*, 427, 344-347.

Enserink M. (2006) Massive Outbreak Draws Fresh Attention to Little – Known Virus, *Science,* 311, P.1085.

Epstein, Paul R, 2006, 'Climate Change and Public Health: Focusing on Emerging Infectious Diseases', Smart Growth and Climate Change Regional Development, *Infrastructure and Adaptation*.

Garg P, Nag Pal J, Khairnar P, Seneviratne SL, 2008, 'Economic Burden of Dengue Infections in India', *Trans R Society of Tropical Medicine and Hygiene,* 102, pp.570-577

Higgs S, 2006, 'The 2005-06 Chikungunya Epidemics in the Indian Ocean', *Vector Borne Zoonotic Dis*, 6, pp.115-6.

Juana, J.S, Narayana N, Mupimpila C, 2004, 'Estimating Household Expenditure on Malaria Interventions in Western Sierra Leone: A Contingent

Kent, Mary M, Yin Sandra, 2006, 'Controlling Infectious Diseases', *Population Bulletin* Vol.61.issue.2.

Laras K, Sukri N.C, Larasati R.P, Bangs M. J, Kosim R, Djauzi, 2005, 'Tracking the Reemergence of Epidemic Chikungunya Virus in Indonesia', *Trans R soc Tropical Medicine and Hygiene*, 99, PP. 128-41.

Levin, Simon A, 2007, 'Introduction; Infectious Diseases', *Environment and Development Economics*, Vol.12, Issue, 5.

Lindelow, Magnus, 2005, 'The Utilization of Curative Healthcare in Mozambique' Does income Matter?' *Journal of African Economics*, Vol.14, Issue, B.

Mavalanker D, Shastri P, Ramani K V, 2007, 'Chikungunya Epidemic Mortality in India: Lessons from "17th Century Bills of Mortality Still Relevant, Ahmadabad,' *Indian Institute of Management*, WorkingPaper- No 12:2-12.

Mourya D.T, Mishra A.C, 2006, 'Chikungunya Fever' *Lancer*, 368(9531) pp. 186-7.

National Institute of Communicable Disease, 2006, Chikungunya Fever CD Alert 10, New Delhi, (2),pp.6-8.

Outbreak New, 'Chikungunya and Dengue South –West India Ocean', *Weekly Epidemic Record*, 2006, 81, pp. 106-8.

Padbidri V.S,Gnaneswar T.T, 1979, 'Epidemiological Investigations of Chikungunya Epidemic at Barsi', *Microbial Manual*, 23, pp. 445-51.

Powersa M, Broulta C, Tesh R.B, Weaver S.C, 2000, 'Reemergence of Chickungunya and Onyongnuong Viruses: Evidences for districts', *Geographical Lineages and Districts Evolutionary Relationships Environ*, 81, pp. 47-9.

Ravi V, 2006, 'Re-emergence of Chikungunya Virus in India', *Indian Journal of Medical Microbiology*, 24, pp.83-4.

Staikowsky F, Pinar A, Land E, Grivard P, Tallermin F, Michauld A, 2006, 'The Infection by the Virus Chikungunya; An Emergent Disease in the Reunion Island,' *Eur J Emerg med,*13: A, pp. 7-8.

Thiruvengadum K.V, Kalyanasundaram V, Rajgopal J, 1965, 'Clinical and Pathological Studies on Chikungunya Fever in Madras City', *Indian Journal of Medicine*, 53, pp.729-44.

Valuation Approach,' *Journal of International Environment and Development*, Vol-1, Issue 1.

World Health Organisation, 2000, International Conference on Mosquito Control: Recommendations, *Weekly Epidemic Research 2000*, WHO, 75, pp.173-5.

Estimation Of Cost Of Illness Of Infectious Diseases

Introduction

Cost of illness (COI) measures economic burden of a disease or diseases and estimates the amount that could be potentially saved of a disease to be eradicated. The COI studies are instrumental in public health policy debates for taking policy decisions and highlighting the magnitude of an illness. It will also help the policy makers in deciding the priority of health expenditure on health care or prevention policy. The policy makers frequently use COI studies for supplying information of a disease to stakeholders of government. The cost figures from COI studies are used in cost effectives of a particular health expenditure and cost benefit analysis. Cost effectives and cost benefit analyses give additional information not included in the cost studies that used to take best course of action. COI is just one tool of measurement used for health economics. In estimating cost of illness, both indirect and direct costs are often taken into account. The estimate of other social and economic costs due to illness includes loss of production due to sickness or death and imputed cost of non-marketed work.

Perspectives of Cost of Illness Estimation

A COI estimation can be made based on different perspectives. Each of them is made to serve different purpose. The COI estimation based on various perspectives differs. The important perspectives of COI include COI to the society, COI to the health care system, COI to the third party payers, COI to the business, COI to the government and COI to the household or sick person. The purpose of a study decided ultimately the necessary perspective. A COI study concerned with medical care costs would require healthcare system the perspective, a COI study concerned with the government could require the information for the allocation of the expenditure for the health care. It is not necessary that the COI study should take only one perspective.

Outcome Trees

To provide a basis for disease burden and cost-of-illness calculations, the construction of an outcome tree is a useful first step. An outcome tree represents a qualitative representation of the disease progression over time by ordering relevant health states following infection and illustrating their conditional dependency. Constructing outcome trees implies making choices on which outcome or resources are to include and which are to exclude. This is ideally based on systematic literature reviews; however, most infectious diseases are associated with a large number of clinical outcomes, some of which may be rare and / or of limited severity. Deciding which outcomes to include in the tree requires preliminary estimations of:

a) The relative impact of all possible outcomes on the total disease burden and
b) The relative impact of all possible resource requests on the total cost-of-illness.

Depending on the complexity of the outcome tree, the incidence must be assessed for a varying number of non-fatal outcomes. Ideally this task would involve the establishment of the incidence of one outcome at the root of the tree (i.e. acute gastro- enteritis) and the (conditional) probability of progressing to the next stage or to recovery. In practice such data are rarely available for a complete outcome tree and supplementary data are necessary.

The population at Risk

Population attributable risk (PAR), is an epidemiological concept and it defines its role in prevention. Using this concept of PAR, the amount of morbidity and mortality attributable to physical inactivity can be assessed. An estimate made of the fraction of disease that might be prevented if the population became more active. This concept is useful for defining the health benefits of regular moderate activity.

Risk of disease are often assessed by comparing rates of health or disease in some groups exposed to a risk factor, compared to those not exposed to the risk factor, for example, those who smoke tobacco are more than ten times likely to develop lung cancer, compared to non-smokers. This is usually described as a relative risk (the ratio of rates of disease or outcome) in the exposed group as compared to those unexposed to the risk. The relative risk is a measure of the strength of association between exposure and outcome.

Absolute comparisons between groups are described in terms of attributable risks. The risk difference which is also known as the excess absolute risk is the difference between rates of outcome experienced by groups who are exposed and unexposed to relative risk factors. When this concept is expressed for the whole population it is known as the population attributable risk (PAR). This is defined as the proportion of a given health outcome attributable to a risk factor in the population. Using the relative risks derived from epidemiological studies, and the prevalence of physical inactivity, the population attributable risk (PAR) can be calculated. This percentage of deaths or any outcome in a population that could be attributed to inactivity should, strictly speaking, be called the PAR fraction, or attributable fraction, as it represents a percentage of the outcome attributable to exposure.

This measure is useful for assessing the public health importance of risk factors, as it represents the proportion of cases or deaths (or other outcomes) prevented if exposure to the risk factor were eliminated (Bauman 1998). Two factors contribute the magnitude of the PAR prevalence and the strength of association. Note that higher prevalence of inactivity in the population, or a stronger association between inactivity and a health outcome will both result in a greater PAR. The formula for the population attributable risk (PAR) is shown below where:

P = Prevalence of inactivity in the population and
RR = Relative risk (of outcome) in the sedentary / low activity group
    compared with the active group.
Population attributable risk= P (RR-1) / 1 + P (RR – 1)

Using the formula above, some examples are described below assume that P, the population prevalence of physical inactivity is 0.5 (around 50 percent inactive) and the relative risk for the relationship between inactivity and incident coronary heart disease (CHD) is estimated to be around 1.9 (From Berlin 1990)

Then the PAR = 0.5 (1.9 – 1) / 1 + 0.5 (1.9 – 1) = 0.31

The prevalence of inadequate physical activity is the community especially amongst older adult and the strength of association between inactivity and specific disease. Mortality and morbidity would indicate substantial health sector resources are used in the diagnosis and treatment of preventable disease.

Types of Cost of Illness Studies

COI studies estimate the economic burden of a particular disease upon the society. The COI studies used to analyse either prevalence or incidence costs. The prevalence based studies determine the costs incurred by all individuals with the disease during a defined period, usually one year. The costs are usually categorised as direct or indirect. In the case of direct medical costs, the sources of major expenses (i.e., inpatient outpatient, health care providers and drugs) are to be identified.

1. Incidence Based Studies

An incidence – based analysis estimates the cost for each patient recently diagnosed with the disease within a defined period. This type of analysis utilises the progression of the disease to estimate its lifetime costs. The focus of this method is health care expenditure for the lifetime of the patient. It is not an appropriate method for diseases with a long survival time. The estimated values of preventive measures often utilise the results of incidence based analyses.

Incidence-based studies, which estimate lifetime costs, measure the costs of an illness from the onset to the conclusion of a disease. Incidence costs include the discounted lifetime medical, morbidity, and mortality costs for the incident cohort.

The incident based COI studies estimates life time cost of an illness from the onset to the conclusion. Chikungunya fever is not fatal and recovery from the fever is not more than two weeks from the onset of illness. The significant part of the disease is the severe losing of productivity and working day lose after the recovery. This period is also not the same for victims of Chikungunya fever. Some of them changed their occupation involving less physical exertion. Another important phase is the side effects due to Chikungunya fever. The side effects are often in association with immunity of the person to withstand the fever or type of treatment and nature of job pursued. Thus the incidence cost of Chikungunya fever includes discounted medical cost and the morbidity and mortality cost of the incident cohort.

2. Prevalence Based Studies

Prevalence based studies, which estimate annual costs, measure the COI in one period usually a year, regardless of the date of onset. The prevalence based study includes all medical cost and morbidity cost of a disease in a year. However, mortality cost and disability cost of the prevalence based studies are estimated differently from the other costs, the prevalence based studies are more common because they require less data and fever assumption.

The methods of calculating life time costs using annual cost data differ; however, each method uses annual data as a cross section of how costs are distributed by age. The assumption is that the cross sectional views of the cost at different ages represent the progression of the disease. One of the methods to estimate the difference in cost incurred by those with the disease and those without disease is by age group. It provides per capita incremental cost by age for those with the disease which can include data on the number of people with disease who are expected to survive in each age to set the life time cost estimate. Another method used to estimate the life time cost is by combining the annual unit cost data with the expert opinion about the course of disease. It can also estimate on the basis of the percentage of cost incurred in the first year for a related condition. Averting the cost approach is also useful in cost effectiveness analysis. The cost benefit analysis for an illness prevention of an acute illness, a prevalence based or incidence based approach would yield the same result because illness has cost within one year or there exist no future cost. The cost of illness of Chikungunya fever falls heavily on the poor because the direct and indirect cost of the disease often represents a significant the proportion of the household income. Although COI theoretically includes the cost of pain and suffering, it is generally excluded from calculation because of its difficulty. A better approach to include the tangible costs is the WTP approach, which originally designed to assign values of public goods. Such values are subjected to personal interpretation and biased because the respondents interest to engage in strategic behaviour. This problem can be avoided by carefully constructed survey with closed ended questions. The COI approach fails to account for lost productivity in the event, when patient return to work before fully recovered from Chikungunya.

Components of Total Cost of Illness

COI studies include both direct and indirect cost. The direct cost measure the opportunity cost of resources used for treating a particular disease, where as indirect cost measure the value of resources loss due to particular illness. Some studies also include intangible cost of paying and suffering on the form quality of life measure. This is omitted in many studies because of the difficulty in accurately quantifying it in monetary term.

Cost Categories of Total Cost of Illness

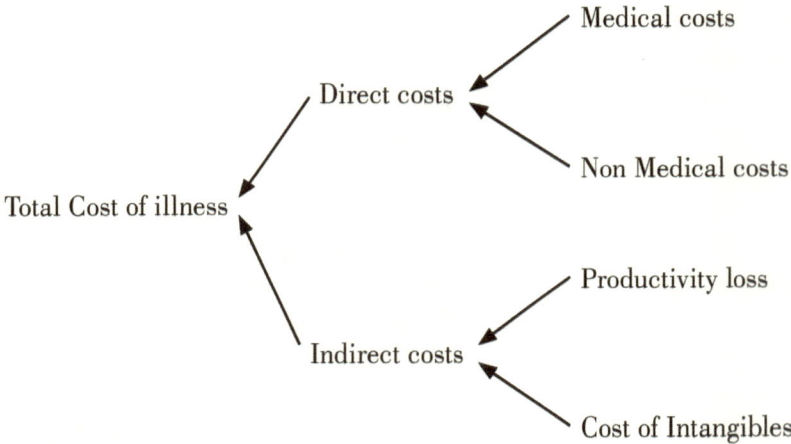

Cost of illness can also be calculated by adding of direct health care costs (DHC) and indirect -health care costs (DNHC) and direct and indirect non-health care costs (INHC).

Cost of Illness = Direct Health Care Costs + Indirect Health Care Costs + Direct Non-Health Care Costs + Indirect Non-Health Care Costs.

The units of analyses in the COI are not unique. Generally cost per illness episode, per capita cost of illness or household cost of illness are the common approaches used for the computation of COI. Among these approaches, cost of illness per household is preferred as a unit of analysis for assessing the economic costs of illness. The economic consequences of illness in the form of expenditure decisions and source of finance for treatment are based on negotiations and policy of resources within the household. The COI rarely fall on the sick person but on other household members who finance and care for the sick and accompany them to get treatment. Moreover COI fall on the household budget which has implications of the resources available for other uses and for other members (Berman et al., 1994; Sanerborn et al., 1995).

A) Direct Costs

Direct costs of illness refer to all household expenditure linked with seeking and obtaining treatment including medical and non-medical expenses such as transport or special foods.

Direct medical costs consist of costs incurred by the health care system during the delivery of medical care. This includes costs associated with hospitalisation and nursing home stay. Health care providers, drugs, laboratory tests and outpatient procedures such as outpatient surgery, physical therapy and occupational therapy are dependent on the perspectives used for the analysis. Direct non-medical costs may also be included in the direct costs. These costs include the patient's out of pocket expenditure, home care provided by family members and expenditures associated with the transportation of patients to receive medical care.

Direct medical cost are the summation of hospital inpatient, physician inpatient physician outpatient, emergency department, outpatient nursing home care, hospital care, specialists and other professionals care, diagnostic tests, drugs and drug sundries and medical supplies.

For each health outcome of a specific disease and for each specific medical service, the direct health care costs related to a specific pathogen are estimated by multiplying the number of cases requiring health care service (m) by the required health care service unit per case (p) and by the costs per health care service unit (mc). The formula for direct health care costs for a specific pathogen for health outcome and for health care service is in basic notation.

$$DHC = \sum_{1} (\sum_{1} m_{1} X P_{1} X mC_{1})$$

The important difficulty in calculating direct medical costs, particularly the hospital cost is that the households remember almost the exact total hospital cost of the Chikungunya episodes in the household. But it is difficult for them to give the exact amount in each component of the direct medical cost and the medical expenditure of each victim of Chikungunya in a household. Repeated discussions on the history of episode often reveal the important expenses of direct costs. Hence the assessment of direct medical cost is not an overestimation of the COI. To obtain more accurate estimates, information are obtained from specific hospitals, doctors and medical centres about centres about the charges doctors and medical centres used to charge for various components of direct costs.

i) Direct Non-Health Care Costs

Travel costs of patients, costs for additional diapers, and co-payments by patients for medicines, informal care etc, are some examples of direct non-health care costs. For each health outcome (i) of a specific disease and for each specific non-health care services, the direct non-health care costs related to a specific pathogen were estimated by multiplying the number of cases requiring non-health care services (r) by the required non-health care service units per case (q) and by the costs per non-health care service unit (rc). The formula for direct non-health care costs for a specific pathogen for health outcome r and for non-health care service j is in basic notation.

$$DNHC = \sum_i \left(\sum_i r_i \times q_i \times rc_{j)} \right)_i$$

Non medical direct cost includes transportation cost to various health care centres by the members of a household while giving treatment for a disease. Many of the non-medical direct cost may not be included in the COI estimation.

B) Indirect Cost

Indirect COI are defined as the loss of productive labour time due to illness, for both patients and caregivers. The scope of indirect costs included in the COI studies varies (Chime et al., 2003). The indirect costs include time spent on seeking treatment to the patients and opportunity cost of time lost to caregiver. Some studies go further and measure the opportunity cost of mortality in terms of lifetime income foregone.

The cost related to productivity loss attributable to a disease and its treatment is indirect costs. Some diseases primarily affect age groups who are active participants in the labour workforce. For those diseases the indirect costs comprise a larger percentage of the total COI. The indirect costs associated with diseases related to elderly people are usually less important because they are not in the working age group. Another category of indirect costs is intangible costs, which reflect a patient's weightage on pain and suffering. It is difficult to quantify the monetary value of these costs resulting in the omission of intangible costs in most of the COI analysis.

Indirect Health Care Costs

Indirect health care costs comprise future savings in health care costs in the life years lost due to premature death. The total indirect health care costs are estimated by accounting the costs for different medical services. For each health outcome of a specific disease and for each specific medical service, the direct health care costs related to a specific pathogen are estimated by multiplying the number of cases requiring health care service (m) by the required health care service unit per case (p) and by the costs per health care service unit (mc). The formula for indirect health care costs for a specific pathogen for health outcome and for health care service is in basic notation.

$$IHC = = \sum_1 \sum_1 M_1 X \ P_1 xmc_1)$$

i) Indirect Non-Health Care Costs (INHC)

Indirect non-health care costs, which are defined as the value of production lost to society due to the disease.

a) Temporary absence from work
b) Permanent or long-term disability, and
c) Premature mortality

The estimation of productivity losses includes not only sick persons but also that of the caretakers. The indirect non-health care costs for a specific pathogen are estimated for each health outcome (l) of a specific disease and for each type of sickness leave (k) separately by multiplying the number cases with sickness leaves (s) by the duration of sickness leaves (u) by the wage costs (v) per day. The formula for indirect non-health care costs for a specific pathogen for health outcome and for each episode of sickness leave k are in basic notation.

$$INHC = \sum_1 \left(\sum_1 s_k \ x \ u_k \ x \ v_k \right)_1$$

D) Health Care Payments

There are four possible categories of health care payments.

1) Direct health care costs paid by health insurance and public health authorities;
2) Indirect health care costs paid by health insurances and public health authorities
3) Costs paid by patients themselves; and
4) Indirect costs paid by other stakeholders in the society other than health insurance, public health authorities or the patients.

The first category includes the valuation for medical services such as general practice (GP) consultations, specialist consultation, hospitalization, drugs, rehabilitation and other medical services associated with the patients.

Travel costs of patients, informal care, adjusting houses for disabled patients, and other co-payments paid by patients are some of the examples of costs that are directly related to illness. But this cost occurs outside the health care sector, and are mostly paid by the patients themselves or by social security plans.

The fourth category of costs occur in other sectors most of which occur indirectly related to the illness. Productivity losses due to work absence of patients and care takers of sick people are the main categories of costs in this category. Production losses are due to the temporary absence from work, permanent long-term disability and or premature mortality. Apart from productivity loss, the costs for special education or re-education after having been disabled due to illness, costs for monitoring and follow up of outbreak are also included in this category.

Measurement of Cost Components

Direct costs can be estimated by using any one of the three approaches, the top-down approach, the bottom-up approach, or the econometric approach.

Top–Down Approach

The top-down approach is also known as the epidemiological or attributable risk approach that measures the exposure of a disease or risk factors. The approach uses aggregated data along with a Population Attributable Fraction (PAF) to calculate attributable costs. Cost of Illness studies often use an epidemiological measure which Morgenstern and others used. In this approach, the proportion of medical care for disease B attributable to disease A is measured as follows:

$$PAF = P(RR\text{-}1) / [P(RR\text{-}1) + 1]$$

Where P is the prevalence rate of disease A and RR is the unadjusted relative risk of disease B for people with disease A, compared with those without disease A. However, this equation applies only in limited cases where other factors do not affect the association between diseases A and B.

Generally in COI determination, confounding variables such as age, sex and other similar variables may influence people with disease (A) and people without the disease. If the confounding variables are not controlled, it causes usually upward bias in the relative risk. For example, there is an association between diabetes and heart disease yet those with diabetes and heart disease tend to be high when people become older. The COI fail to account for age when calculating the PAF, and then the calculation of PAF would lead to bias. A couple of adjustment methods are available to account for confounding variables when calculating the PAF. Such methods are Mantel – Haenszed approach and the weighted – sum approach. A common error when using the top down approach, which can significantly impact the estimates, is the use of a partially adjusted method rather than one of the two methods. The error consists of using the PAF equation which can occur only when used with unadjusted relative risks. The error occurs when studies account for the confounding variables while calculating the relative risks and plugs. These errors adjust relative risks into the PAF equation. This error is exacerbated if effect modification is also present but not accounted for. Similar to confounding, modification effect exists when a third factor affects the association between disease A and group B through interaction.

Bottom – Up Approach

It is clear that potentially more cumbersome methods are needed to prevent bias in the bottom – up approach. Bottom –up approach or econometric approach is an alternative for top-down approach. The bottom-up approach estimates costs with calculating the average cost of treatment of the illness and multiplying it by the prevalence of the illness. Since the average cost of treatment of an illness is seldom readily available, the average cost of treatment in the bottom-up approach is calculated by adding together the various pieces of the cost of treatment. The bottom-up approach calculates average cost of treatment by multiplying the unit cost of a particular treatment with the average amount of utilisation. For example, the average cost of illness of outpatient physician care for a particular illness. The method is repeated for each type of care to obtain the total average cost. It is then multiplied with the prevalence of illness to get an estimate of the total direct costs.

Econometric Approach

The econometric or incremental approach estimates the difference in costs between a cohort of the population with the disease and a cohort of the population without the disease. The two cohorts are usually matched, by a regression analysis, using various demographic characteristics and other illness characteristics as independent variables. Within the econometric approach, there are two methods, one by using a mean differences approach and the other by a multi – stage regression approach. The mean differences approach compares the mean costs incurred by each of the two cohorts to determine the incremental difference attributable to the disease of interest.

A multi-stage regression is typically run if there are a large number of cases with zero costs and a few cases with very high cost. The incremental cost of the disease is measured by comparing the regression estimate with the disease dummy variable turned on to the regression estimate with the disease dummy variable turned off. The multiple-stage regression often uses a two-stage regression in the cost estimation, although there are varieties of multiple stage regression. The approach involves estimating the likelihood of an individual receiving any care and then the excess cost of care if recovered. Because the econometric approach measures the incremental difference between persons who have the disease and those who do not. The top-down approach usually requires data on the costs as well as on the relative risks. The bottom-up approach often requires data from multiple sources for the unit cost and utilisation rate of the different types of care.

Low income countries have a large working population engaged in rural and informal sector which limits the effective taxation capacity of the governments. In middle-income and upper-income countries, large segments of the work force engaged in urban and the formal sectors, and it is relatively easy to tax workers at source and design health care systems. In most of the low-income countries, the proportion formal employment is small relative to the informal employment. In these countries a majority of the population receive health care benefits is through effective collective arrangements to obtain protection from health cost.

Faced with overwhelming demand and very limited resources, many governments find it difficult to ration health care services targeted on the poor. In many low-income countries, the rich often benefit more than the poor from public subsidies and public expenditure on health care. The poorest of the poor and socially excluded groups were often not included in community – based initiatives for financing health care. A majority of the people does not benefit from formal insurance coverage, and government expenditure often fails to meet the basic health needs of the poor. The user charges for health care add significantly to the financial hardship of poor households which are often exposed to the reason for indebtedness. Health care costs are not uniform and they differ widely among the different sources.

B. Measurement of Indirect Costs

I. Human Capital Methods

The human capital approach is the most common method used for calculating indirect costs of an illness. One of the important criticisms levelled against this approach is that certain groups are assigned higher values than others. Since human capital approach uses wage rates and employment rates for calculating indirect cost of illness, classification of people in terms of age, sex or race earns less and therefore consequently assigned lower value.

The human capital approach often includes the value of household work, usually valued as the opportunity cost of hiring and replacement of the sick persons in the labour market.

II. Life Time Cost and Productivity Loss

Lifetime costs can be calculated from annual costs, assuming a steady state of disease incidence, progression, survival rate and treatment. But the estimates may not be as accurate as using actual longitudinal data on the full course of the illness. It is because of potential future changes in medical care technology and other assumptions. Despite this limitation, numerous methods provide useful approximations of lifetime costs using annual data, all of which involve the assumption that the structure of future costs is the same as the structure of current costs and then discounting future costs.

For measuring productivity loss, both human capital approach and the friction cost approach are used. The human capital approach is based on neoclassical labour theory. The value of loss of production due to illness is as a consequence of permanent disability or premature death at a specific expected life time. The total productivity starting from that age until the age of retirement is counted as productivity losses. The aim of the friction cost approach is to adjust the human capital estimates of productivity costs for compensations. The friction cost method considers only production losses for the replacement of a sick, invalid or dead worker in the 'friction period. The friction cost method takes into account the economic processes by which a sick or a dead person is replaced after a period of adaptation. The length of the friction period depends on the labour market. For instance, a high unemployment rate generally allows fast replacement of a sick or dead person whereas in the case of a low unemployment rate, more time is needed for replacement. This method places a zero value on persons outside the labour market, such as children and aged. Illness attributable to physical inactivity is an important issue for health care providers, policy makers and communities. The friction cost method measures the production losses to the replacement of a worker. This approach assumes short-term work losses made up by an employee. The loss or absence of an employee results in additional costs time of hiring and training a new employee. The cost of hiring an employee to fully given training is known as the friction period.

Human Capital Vs Friction Cost

The human capital method of COI is mainly criticised because of overvaluing indirect costs. The friction cost methods claims that the productivity losses are often eliminated after a new employee is trained and replaced. However, the friction cost method is rarely used because it requires extensive data to estimate the losses in the friction period. The productivity loss is not unique. There are several categories of loss of productivity. Work absenteeism of an individual due to morbidity results in lost wages per individual if paid sick days are not available: When paid sick days are available, then the cost of absenteeism is not included under indirect costs because it is borne by the employer. The second category of productivity loss is loss of efficiency. It results from the inability of the individual to work at full capacity or when the individual assumes the responsibilities of a lower level job because of the inability to work efficiently in the current job, when compared to his performance in the same job before the infliction of the disease.

There are two areas of controversy exist with regard to the inclusion of indirect costs in the estimation of COI. First controversy is about the inclusion of indirect costs in the COI analysis and the second is about the suitability of methods used for measuring the indirect non-medical costs. Proponents advocate the inclusion of indirect costs maintain that exclusion of these costs result in underestimation of the true COI. Critics of indirect costs insist the exclusion of indirect costs because these costs are irrelevant to decision-making. The comparison of COI is easier without indirect costs; therefore indirect costs are often indistinguishable for policy making. Moreover, indirect costs calculation is frequently difficult requiring a lot of time and resources. The cost of the same physical level of intangibles shows different cost to different patients.

The second controversy is related to the identification of valuation method appropriate for indirect non-medical costs. The common methods used for calculating indirect costs include human capital approach and the friction cost method. The human capital approach estimates indirect costs by using potential productivity loss valued in terms of potentially lost earnings. This method is based on earnings and it assumes wages as accurately as a measure economic value. A frequent criticism of this method is that it gives greater weight to certain groups. Because of their relative earnings, greater weight is being given to men when compared to women, middle-aged compared to the young and elderly and those who receive compensation for their work compared to those who do not receive compensation, which includes home makers and volunteers. This differential weighting may also have ethical consideration if the inclusion of indirect costs supports the use of medical interventions primarily among individuals of the work force.

Critics of this method contend that for short-term absences may not affect the work because usually co-workers complete an individual's work of an absentee due to illness or the individual will complete the work after they return to work after illness. In the case of long-term absences, replacements will be made for unemployed people. Thus a long absence from work will not have much impact on society but it will seriously impact the sick individual. The potential loss of earning on the part of the COI uses the human capital approach that frequently produces inflated values.

The basis of the friction cost method of evaluation of cost of productivity associated with a disease is the length of time an organization needs to restore its initial level of production and costs. It assumes that losses in productivity always occur to some degree, but the amount of loss is dependent on the time required to replace the sick workers or to reorganise the production process.

The availability of qualified individuals within the organisation and the current unemployment rate influences this length of time. If unemployment decreases, the time required to fill vacancies will increase resulting in higher costs during the period of adaptation or friction period. Production decreases or remains constant at higher costs during the friction period; indirect costs are proportional to the length of the adaptation period. The important disadvantage of this method is that the time period used to calculate the cost is organisation specific and an analysis conducted other than at an organisation level is burdensome.

Controversy exists with regard to the inclusion of various cost components under indirect costs. There are also differences of opinion related to the mere inclusion of indirect costs in the estimation of COI. The calculation of indirect cost by using the human capital approach values potential loss in productivity in terms of loss of earnings. The friction cost method estimates indirect cost by measuring the length of time a particular organisation takes to return its initial production and cost.

C. Willingness to Pay Method

The willingness to pay (WTP) approach measures the amount an individual would be willing to pay for reducing the probability of getting illness or mortality. There are various methods available for determining an individual's WTP. It includes additional wages for jobs with high risks and higher demand for products that lead to greater health or safety.

The WTP approach usually assigns higher value of life than the human capital approach. However, this approach is often difficult to implement in COI studies for a specific disease. Extensive surveys of people's preference are needed although the result relies heavily on people's responses to very specific hypothetical questions about their willingness to avoid certain illness. For communicable diseases, surveys may not fully capture the cost of the disease because of the problem of externalities, people account for only cost without accounting the societal benefit of having fewer people in a society with communicable diseases. Thus the willingness to pay method is often not feasible for a cost of illness study of a specific communicable disease.

D. Social Cost of Specific Disease

Economic research has been conducted to estimate the social costs by international institutions like WHO and World Bank to measure the specific diseases to complement the efforts of international bodies' global burden of disease studies.

Quality – Adjusted life – years (QALYs), Disability – Adjusted life – years (DALYs), Disability – Adjusted Life Expectancy (DALE) or Healthy Adjusted Life Expectancy (HALE) are some of the measurements commonly used to compare health status of different countries and health outcomes of policy interventions.

Disability Adjusted Life years (DALY) measures several possible health outcomes ranging from acute self-limiting disease to chronic disabilities or even mortality into a single composite monetary measure. The DALY is a health gap measure that measures the potential years of life lost due to sickness. Health cost is the total amount of money expended to derive utility from health care services.

Health cost at the household level is the direct and indirect cost incurred to a household as a result of the health problems of some of its members. It includes out of pocket costs and implicit cost (indirect cost) excluding the social cost premature death or years of healthy life lost in the states of less than full-health or disability. According to the WHO, DALY is described as:

DALY = YLL +YLD
YLL = Number of years of life lost due to mortality;
YLD =Number of years lived with disability. It is weighted with a factor between O and 1.

Infectious diseases typically have several possible health outcomes ranging from acute self-limiting diseases to chronic disabilities or even mortality. The different outcome can be combined in single composite measures such as the Disability Adjusted Life Years (DALY). The disease burden and cost-of-illness calculations need to make several choices.

Disability Adjusted Life Years (DALY)

The DALY is a health gap measure that extends the potential years of life lost due to premature death which is equivalent to years of healthy life lost in states of less than full health. One DALY is equal to loss of one year of healthy life (WHO definition). The DALY has been described by Murray and others as:

DALY = YLL + YLD.

YLL is the number of years of life lost due to mortality and YLD is the number of years lived with a disability weighted with a factor ranging between 0and1 representing zero disability and represents on the value of one shows maximum severity of disability. The YLL due to a specific disease in a specified population is calculated by the summation of the cost of all fatal cases. (0) YLL is the health outcome of a specific diseases, each mortaring case multiplied by the expected individual life span of each case (e) at the age of death. Thus

$$YLL = \sum_l n_l x\ t_l x W_l$$

YLL are often an important component of the total disease burden. Lost productivity due to premature death can be an important component of the total cost-of-illness, especially if the human capital approach is applied. Information on the age at death and the life expectancy of fatal cases is important when estimating the productivity losses. The indirect health care costs would remain till the total life years if the illness is not fatal.

8. Difficulties in the Estimation of Cost of Illness

The estimation of COI for individuals and households is fraught with difficulties because of the use of different definitions of cost, different methodologies to measure and quantify cost and different units of analysis (Clima et al.,2003; Mclntyre and Thiede 2003; Worrall et al., 2002).

9. Uses of Cost of Illness Analysis

The estimation of COI is necessary for resource allocation between alternative activities and to select optimum policy mix of curative, preventive and promotive activities. The economic burden of a disease is based on the assessment of social and household cost of morbidity and mortality. Estimates of COI indicate the burden of disease; provide insight into the best alternative use of limited resources.

10. Enveloping a Better Estimate of COI

A substantial improvement could be made in the COI studies by eliciting the best available information, rather than using lower bound estimates. Another method of improvement is to take a more explicit approach to deal with uncertainty by simulation and the development of estimation ranges.

Morbidity related productivity effects can be estimated through regression analyses of household health survey data, and the socio, economic and demographic factors associated with the household. The productivity losses can be valued with respect to age specific labour earning and household production function. The COI includes productivity losses associate with illness and premature death; and are typically measured as the value of lost productivity to an individual or household due to illness.

11. Conclusion

The cost of illness estimation at the household level is useful in understanding the intensity of the disease among different sections of the society. Moreover, the different components of the cost of illness is not uniform for different diseases especially the communicable disease. Hence the weight of direct and indirect costs and the order of priority will be useful for taking optimal policy decisions.

REFERENCES

Abel-Smith B, Rawal P, 1994, 'Employer's Willingness to Pay: The Case for Compulsory Health Insurance in Tanzania', *Health Policy and Planning,* 9(4), pp.409-18.

American Diabetes Association, 'Economic Costs of Diabetes in the U S in 2002'. *Diabetes Care 2003*, 26(3),pp.917-932.

Barger K, Ehlken B, Kugland B, Augustin M, 2005, 'Cost of Illness in Patients with Moderate and Severe Chronic Psoriasis Vulgar in Germany' *J Dtsch Dermatology Ges*, 3 p511-8.

Bartlett J.C, Miller L.S, Rice D.P, Max W, 1994, 'Medical Care Expenditures Attributable to Cigarette Smoking – United States', *Morbidity Mortality weekly Report,* 43 pp.469-472.

Benichou J A, 2001, 'Review of Adjusted Estimators of Attributable Risk', *Statistical Methods in Medical Research*,10(3), pp.195-216.

Bloom B S, Bruno D J, Maman D y, and Jayadevappa R, 2001 'Usefulness of US Cost of Illness Studies in Healthcare Decision Making, *Pharmacoeconpmics*, 19(2), pp.207-213.

Briggs A, 1999, 'Handling Uncertainty in Economic Evaluation' *B M J*, 319(7202), P.120.

Cohen D R and Henderson J B, 1988, 'Health Prevention and Economics', Oxford University press.

Cooper B S and Rice D P, 1976, 'The Economic Cost of Illness Revisited', *Social Security Bulletin*, 39(2), pp.21-36.

Currie G, kerfoot K D, Donaldson C, and Macarthur C, 2006, 'Are Cost of Injury Studies Useful?', *Injury Prevention*, 6, pp.175-176.

Drummond M, 1992, 'Cost-of-illness Studies; A Major Headache?', *Pharmacoeconomics*, 2(1), pp.1-4.

Drummond. M F,1997, Et al (eds), 'Methods for the Economic Evaluations of Health Care Programmers', 2nd Edition, Oxford University Press.

Finkelstein E.A, Fiebelkorn I.C, and Wang G, 2003, 'National medical spending Attributable to Overweight and obesity: How Much and who's paying', *Health Affairs*, 14 may: 219, w3 P.226.

Finkler S A, 1982, 'The Distinction between Costs and Charges', *Annals of Internal Medicine*, 96, pp.102-109.

Flegal K M, Graubard B I, Williamson D F, and Gail M H, 2005, 'Excess Deaths Associated with Underweight, Overweight, and Obesity', *JAMA*, 293 (115), pp.1861-1867.

Flegal K M, Graubard B I, and Williamson D F, 2004, 'Methods of Calculating Deaths Attributable to Obesity', *American Journal of Epidemiology*, 160(4), pp.331-338.

Ford S, Torgerson D J, Raftery J,2000, 'Cost of Illness Studies', *BMJ*, 320, P.1335.

Freedberg K A, Scharfstein J A, Seage G R III, L osina E, Weinstein M C, Craven D E, and paltiel A D,1998, 'The Cost-Effectiveness of Preventing AIDS-Related Opportunistic Infections', *JAMA*, 279(2), pp.130-136.

French M T and Martin R F, 1996, 'The Costs of Drug Abuse Consequences'-A Summary of Research Findings', *Journal of Substance Abuse Treatment*, 13(6),pp.453-466.

Gallup J, Sad us J, 2001, 'The Economic Burden of Malaria', *Am J Trop Med Hyg,* 64 (Suppl), pp.85-96.

Goetzel R. Z, Long S.R, Ozminkowski R.J, Hawkins K, Wang S, Lynch W, 2004, 'Health Absence, Disability, and Presenteeism Cost Estimates of Certain Physical and Mental Health Conditions Affecting U S Employers'. *Journal of Occupational and Environmental Medicine*, 46, pp.398-412.

Gold M R, Siegel J E, Russell L B, and Weinstein M C, 1996, 'Cost Effectiveness in Health and Medicine', Oxford University Press, New York.

Guhan S, 1994, 'Social Security Options for Developing Countries', *International Labour Review*, 133(1), pp.35-53.

Hodgson T A and Cai L, 2001, 'Medical Care Expenditure for Hypertension, its Complications and its Co Morbidities', *Medical care*, 39(6), pp.599-615.

Hodgson T A and Cohen A J, 1999, 'Medical Care Expenditures for Diabetes, its Chronic Complications, and its Co Morbidities', *Preventive Medicine*,29, pp.173-186.

Hodgson T A and Miners M R, 1982, 'Cost of Illness Methodology; A Guide to Current Practices and Procedures', *Milbank memorial fund Quarterly*, 60(3), pp.429-462.

Hodgson T A, 1982, 'Annual Cost of Illness Versus Lifetime Costs of Illness and Implications of Structural Change', *Drug Information Journal of Public Health*, 72(6), pp.536-538.

Hodgson T A, 1983, 'The State of the Art of Cost of Illness Studies', *Advances in Health Economics and Health Services Research*, 4, pp.129-164.

Hodgson T A, 1994, 'Costs of Illness in Cost-Effectiveness Analysis: A Review of the Methodology', *Pharmacoeconomics*, 6(6), pp.536-552.

Jamison D T, 1993, Et al (eds), 'Disease Control Priorities in Developing Countries, Oxford University Press, New York.

Javitz H S, Ward M M, Watson J B, and Jana M, 2004, 'Cost of Illness of Chronic Angina', *The American Journal of Managed Care*, 10(11Suppl), pp.S358-S369.

Johannesson M and Karlsson G, 1996, *Journal of Health Economics,* 16, pp.249-255.

Koopmanschap M A and Van Ineveld B M, 1992, 'Towards a New Approach for Estimating Indirect Costs of Disease', *Social Science and Medicine*, 34(9), pp.1005-1010.

Landefeld J S and Seskin E P, 1982, 'The Economic Value of Life: Linking Theory to Practice', *American Journal of Public Health*, 72(6), pp.555-566.

Lazar M.A, 2005, 'How Obesity Causes Diabetes: Not a Fall Tale', *Science,* 307(5708), pp. 373-375.

Liu JL, Maniadakis N, Gray A, and Rayner M, 2002, 'The Economic Burden of Coronary Heart Disease in the U K', *Heart*, 88(6), pp. 597-603.

Lowell B, Schulman G.I, 2005, 'Mitochondrial Dysfunction and Type 2 Diabetes', *Science*, 307(5708) pp.384-387.

Luce B.R, Manning W.G, Siegel J.E, and Lipscomb J, 1996, 'Estimating Costs in cost Effectiveness Analysis' in Gold M.R, Siegel J.E, Russell L.B, et al., (eds.), *Cost- effectiveness in Health and medicine*, Oxford University Press, New York.

Macroeconomics and Health, November 3, 2001, 'Investing in Health for Economic Development Geneva, *World Health Organization*.

Mark T L, Woody G E, Juday T, and Kleber H D, 2001, 'The Economic Costs of Heroin Addiction in the United States', *Drug and Alcohol Dependence*,61, pp.195-206.

Miller L.S, Zhang X, Novotny T, Rice D.P, and Max W, 1998, 'State Estimates of Medicaid Expenditures Attributable to cigarette Smoking', Fiscal year 1993, *Public Health Reports*, 113(2) pp.140-151.

Mishan E J, 1971, 'Evaluation of Life and Limb: A Theoretical Approach', Journal of Political Economy, 79(4), pp.687-705.

Morganstern H, Klein Baum D G, and Kupper L L, 1980, 'Measures of Diseases Incidence Used in Epidemiological Research', *International Journal of Epidemiology*, 9, pp.97-104.

Pagano E, Brunetti M, Tediosi F, and Garattini L,1999, 'Costs of Diabetes: A Methodological Analysis of the Literature' *Pharmacoeconomics*, 15(6), pp.583-595.

Reynaud M, Gaudin-Colombel AN F, and Le Pen C, 2001, 'Two Methods of Estimating Health Costs Linked to Alcoholism in France (With a Note on Social Costs)', *Alcohol and Alcoholism,* 36(1), pp.89-95.

Rice D P, 1967, 'Estimating the Cost of Illness American Journal of Public Health, 57(3), pp. 424-440.

Rice D P, 2000, 'Cost of illness Studies: What is Good about Them?' *Injury Prevention*, 6:177-179.

Rice D P, Fox P J, Max W, Webber P A, Lindeman D A, Hauck W, and Segura E, 1993, 'The Economic Burden of Alzheimer's Disease Care', *Health Affairs*, 12(2),pp.164-176.

Rice D P, Kelman S, Miller L S, and Dunmeyer S,1990, 'The Economic Costs of Alcohol and Drug Abuse and Mental Illness', 1985, Rockville, M D: *National institute on Drug Abuse*.

Rice D, 1999, The Economic Burden of Musculoskeletal Conditions, U S, 1995, in Praemer A, Furner S, and Rice D.P (eds), Musculoskeletal Condition in the U S Rosemont, I.L, *American Academy of Orthopedic Surgeons*.

Rice D.P, Mackenzie E.J, 1989, 'Associate Cost of Injury in the United States: A Report to Congress, San Francisco, *C A: Institute for Health and Aging*, Johns Hopkins University.

Rockhill B, Newman B, and Weinberg C, 1998, 'Use and Misuse of Population Attributable Fractions', *American Journal of Public Health*, 88(1), pp.15-19.

Rogowski J, 1999, 'Measuring the Cost of Prenatal and Parental care', *Pediatrics*, 103(suppl 1 E), pp.329-335.

Rothermich EA and Pathak D S, 1999, 'Productivity Cost Controversies in Cost-Effectiveness Analysis: Review and Research Agenda', *Clinical Therapeutics*, 21(1), pp.255-267.

Roux L and Donaldson C, 2004, 'Economics and Obesity: Costing the Problems or Evaluating Solutions?', *Obesity Research*, 12, P.1189.

Sach S J, Warner A, 1995, 'Economic Reform and the Process of Global Integration Brookings Papers', *Econ Activity*, 1, pp. 1-118.

Sachs J, Malancy P, 2002, 'The Economic and Social Burden of Malaria', *Nature,* 415, pp.680-685.

Schieber G, maeda A, 1997, 'Curmudgeon's Guide to Health Care Financing in Developing Countries, Schieber G, editor, 'Innovations in health care financing', Washington (DC), World Bank 1997, 'Proceedings of a World Bank Conference', 10-11 march.

Taylor D.H, and Sloan F.A, 2000, 'How Much Do Persons with Alzheimer's Disease Cost Medicare?,' *Journal of the American Geriatrics Society*, 48: pp.639-646.

The World Health Report, 2000, 'Health Systems: Measuring Performance Geneva', World Health organization.

Thompson D, Edelsberg J, Kinsey K.L, Oster G,1998, 'Estimated Economic Costs of Obesity to US Businesses', *American Journal of Health Promotion*,13(2), pp.120-127.

Van Ginneken W, 1999, 'Social Security for the Informal Sector: New challenges for the developing Countries', *International Social Security Review*, 52(1), pp.49-69.

Warner K.E, Flodgson T.A, and Carroll C.E, 1999, 'Medical Costs of Smoking in the United States: Estimates, Their Validity and Their implication', *Tobacco Control,* 8, pp. 290-300.

World Bank, 1993, *World Development Report 1993*, 'Investing in Health', Oxford University Press, New York.

World Bank, 1997, 'Sector Strategy for HNP', World Bank, Washington (DC).

Zeller M, Sharma M, 2005. 'Many Borrow, More Save, and all Insure: Implications for Food and Micro- Finance Policy, *Food Policy,* 25(2), pp.143-67.

Socio Economic Characteristics Of Chikungunya Affected Households In Kanyakumari District

T he study was conducted in Vilavancode and Kalkulam Taluk of Kanyakumari District. The study is based on primary data collected through interview schedule with the use of well- structured questionnaire. Many socio economic variables, health indicators and disease surveillance information are collected through the survey method. Adoption of the method is justified by the fact that the clinics and hospitals are without testing facilities in their laboratory to detect Chikungunya cases. Most of the diseases are diagnosed symptomatically by the doctors or some symptoms based on clinical experience. The study is focused on households having members diagnosed of Chikungunya fever. However, the symptoms of Chikungunya overlap with those of Malaria and dengue. On the basis of the medical reports of the hospitals, the population list of the Chikungunya affected households are prepared. From the population, list sample households were drawn.

Multi-stage random samplings technique was adopted to identify the sample households. The sample size was decided as 300, out of which only 258 households gave complete answers to the structured questionnaire in the interview schedule.

Descriptive statistics, frequency table, percentages, ratios and averages are some of the tools employed to analyse the socio - economic characteristics. Individual health status is largely determined by the socio economic characteristics of households. Epidemiological evidences suggest that health is determined at least in part by economic and social connectedness. Economic conditions dramatically affect health, immunity and longevity. Many interactions between economic, social and cultural factors help to determine the influence of these factors on community health. The present chapter attempts to unravel the demographic, social and economic characteristics of the selected households in Kanyakumari District of Tamil Nadu.

Description of the Study Area

Kanyakumari District is the southern tip of both peninsular India and Tamil Nadu. It came into existence in 1956 after merging the area with Tamil Nadu. The district head quarter is at Nagercoil. It is bordered with the State of Kerala in the North West, Tirunelveli district of Tamil Nadu in the North and North East, Arabian Sea in the West, Indian Ocean in the South and Gulf of Mannar in the East.

Kanyakumari is one of the smallest districts in Tamil Nadu with an area of 1648 sq.km. The district has almost the entire ecosystem comprising forests, wetlands, fresh water resources, marines etc. The district was once called the granary of Travancore with hundreds of water bodies and an excellent canal irrigation system. The main agriculture crops include rubber and spice plantations, paddy fields, banana and coconut plantations, besides vegetable and paddy fields.

The district has 62 km seacoast on the Western side and 6 km of coast on the Eastern side. The land from the sea-coast gradually rises up to the Western Ghats. The soil types are Laterite, Red and Alluvial soil and the soil PH is between 4.5 and 8.0. The district has two revenue divisions namely Thucklay and Nagercoil and four Taluks namely, Vilavancode, Kalkulam, Agesteeswarm and Thovalai. The district has favourable agro climatic condition, which is suitable for the cultivation of a variety of crops. There is a distinct variation in the climatic conditions within the district, it gets its rainfall both during the South West (June-September) and North East monsoons (October to the mid of December).

Kanyakumari District accounts for 95 percent of the total production of natural rubber in Tamilnadu. Paddy fields, banana and coconut plantations are found on the plains and valleys near the coast. Paddy, banana, tapioca, cashew, mango and spices are the important agricultural crops. Timber productions, honey collection, rubber, tea, fruits and pepper are some of the forestry land activities with the North West area of the district. The economy of the district is agriculture. Out of the total geographic area, Reserve Forest Area comes to about 30 percent. The district is rich in wildlife and its forests are a veritable trove of biological diversion. Rivers (Dams) and ponds are the important source of irrigation.

As per the 2001 census Kanyakumari District had a favourable sex ratio of 1014. The total male population is 8, 32,269 as compared to the female population of 84, 3765. Hindus and Christians are the two dominant religions constituting 51.27 and 44.47 percentage of the total population respectively.

The current study selected Vilavancode and Kalkulam Taluk. Both the Taluk have a large proportion of the area under rubber cultivation. Water stored in the coconut shell is blamed for the widespread infection of Chikungunya in these Taluk. A sizable area of the district is also under banana cultivation.

The economic cost of health effects of Chikungunya fever at the household level is examined by taking 258 sample households from these two Taluks. The inferences of the socio-economic and environmental characteristic of the households are discussed.

Particulars of the Respondents

For the analytical convenience, the particulars of respondents and the household as a whole are described separately. The respondent of the survey is generally the head of the household or the main bread winner of the family on whom the final decision of the household activities is vested.

Sex

The sex of the respondent is presented in Table 6.1.

Table 6.1: Sex of the respondent

Sex	Frequency	Percentage
Male	206	79.8
Female	52	20.2
Total	258	100.0

One out of every five (20.2 percent) of the sample households having Chikungunya affected members is headed by women. Most of them are either widow or separated from their husbands.

Age

The age distribution of the respondents is shown in Table 6.2.

The age distribution of the respondents revealed that 57 percent of the respondents in 258 households are between the ages of 25 and 50 years. The second highest age group of 50 - 75 years consists of 38.8 percent. Respondents below 25 years and above 75 years form only 2.3 and 1.9 percentages respectively. The age distribution shows that majority of the respondents are in the highly productive stage of the working age.

Table 6.2: Age distribution of the respondents

Age (in years)	Frequency	Percentage
Below 25	6	2.3
25 – 50	147	57.0
50 – 75	100	38.8
75 and above	5	1.9
Total	258	100.0

Marital Status

The marital status of the respondents are classified into married, unmarried, widow or widower and divorced or separated. Generally unmarried respondents are from the households where parents are old. Divorced and separated category of respondents is women who are the victims of both economic and social status. The marital status of the respondents is furnished in Table 6.3.

Table 6.3: Marital status

Marital Status	Frequency	Percentage
Unmarried	8	3.1
Married	232	89.9
Widow/Widower	15	5.8
Divorced/ Separated	3	1.2
Total	258	100.0

Out of the 258 respondents, 89.9 percent are married. Unmarried respondents are the main or the only income earner in a household and the household members totally depend on them for their livelihood. They constitute only 3.1 percent of the households. Divorced or separated respondents are the least group with a share of 1.2 percent. Widow/Widower constitutes 5.8 percent, and most of them are women or aged men.

Educational Status and Level of Education

It is found that 12.8 percent of the 258 respondents are illiterate. The households of illiterate respondents represent that they are from poor social background. The illiterate respondents lack public information and literacy that acts as a barrier to having the knowledge about health improving opportunities, health care information and the role of the physician. The literates behave sensibly by maintaining safe environment, take good nutrition, avoid addiction to habits and follow prudent healthcare. The general observation is that people are very health conscious because only one out of every ten respondent is an illiterate. The educational standard of the literate respondents is presented in Table 6.4.

Table 6.4: Educational standard

Educational standard	Frequency	Percentage
Primary school	57	25.3
Middle school	35	15.6
High school	82	36.4
Higher secondary	24	10.7
Graduates	15	6.7
Post-graduates	8	3.6
Professionals	2	0.9
Others	2	0.9
Total	225	100.0

Figure 6.1: Educational standard of the head of the household

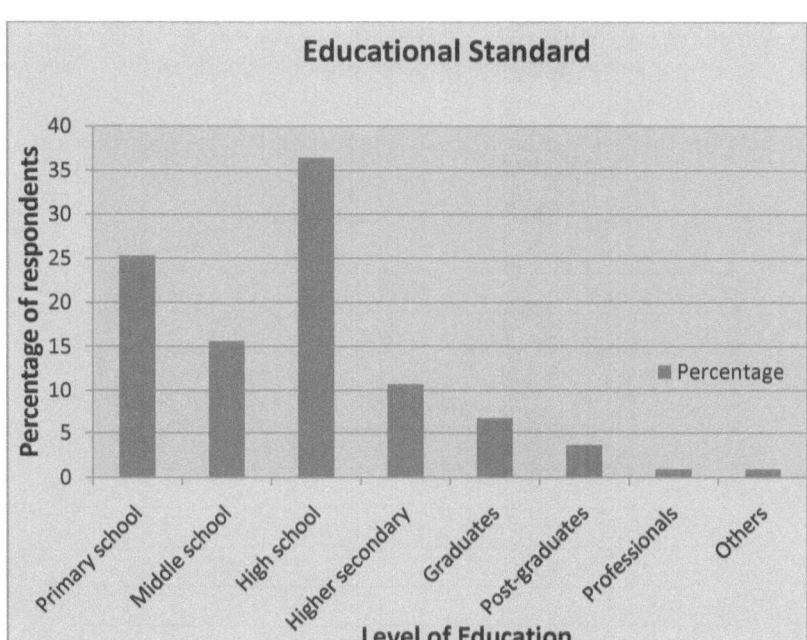

More than one-third (36.4 percent) of the respondents have high school level of education. They form the largest group. The second largest group is respondents educated in the primary school level. It is interesting to note that more than three-fourth (77.3 percent) of the respondents has not crossed the school level of education. Though Kanyakumari District is one of the most literate districts of Tamil Nadu, three out of every four Chikungunya affected household is headed by persons educated up to the school level. Hence it can be concluded that most of the Chikungunya affected households are headed by relatively less educated members with lesser level of educational standard.

Occupation

The occupational pattern of the respondents explains the general socio economic status of a household. Though agriculture is the predominant activity, crops do not require daily employment of people. A major portion of the geographical area selected for the study is under rubber and coconut cultivation. Every household gets some income either directly or indirectly from agriculture. Some households engage in agriculture as a family enterprise because both men and women work in their farm and contribute to the household income. Since labourers are educated they get decent wage. Evidences show that involuntary unemployment is very less among the unskilled labourers.

The occupation pursued by the sample respondents is shown in Table 6.5.

Table 6.5: Occupation

Occupation	Frequency	Percentage
Agriculture	15	5.8
Business	9	3.5
Cashew nut- factory worker	5	1.9
Construction	7	2.7
Driver	7	2.7
Fishing	12	4.7
Government employee	11	4.3
Industrial worker	7	2.7
Mason	7	2.7
Home-making	21	8.1
Tailor	4	1.6
Teacher	7	2.7
Unskilled labourer	128	49.6
Total	258	100.0

It is interesting to note that 49.6 percent of the respondents occupied as unskilled labourers. Many of them work as agricultural labourers, helpers in construction activities and coolies. Female respondents (8.1 percent) take the responsibility of household chores besides engage themselves in some part-time income earning pursuits. Respondents engaged in agricultural activities in their own land represent 5.8 percent. Construction workers, drivers, mason and teachers are 2.7 percent respectively in each category. Respondents in formal employment in the category of soldier, Government employee, and industrial workers are in the percentages of 3.1, 4.3 and 2.7 respectively. The occupational pattern of the respondents reflects that a majority of them are from poor socio- economic background. A majority of the respondents are in the category of informal workers hence absence of employment means no income for them.

Household Characteristics

Households possess certain common characteristics. They include caste, community, religion, mother tongue and type of family.

Caste

The caste composition of the sample households is given in Table 6.6. Nadar caste is the single largest caste representing three fourth (74 percent) of the sample households. But Nadar caste is divided on the basis of religion as Christian Nadars and Hindu Nadars sharing 49.2 and 24.8 percentages respectively. This classification is needed because their culture and lifestyle differ based on their religion. Other dominant caste is the Fishermen who are found in the coastal areas of Arabian Sea. Some of them are found in the hinterland engaged in fish sales activities. They represent 5.8 percent of the sample households. Panickar, Parayar and Mukkudi castes share 3.9, 3.9, and 3.5 percentages respectively of the sample households.

Table 6.6: Caste composition

Castes	Frequency	Percentage
Chekkala	6	2.3
Christian Nadar	127	49.2
Fishermen	15	5.8
Hindu Nadar	64	24.8
Mukkudi	9	3.5
Nair	7	2.7
Panickar	10	3.9
Parayar	10	3.9
Others	10	3.9
Total	258	100.0

Figure 6.2: Castes composition of households

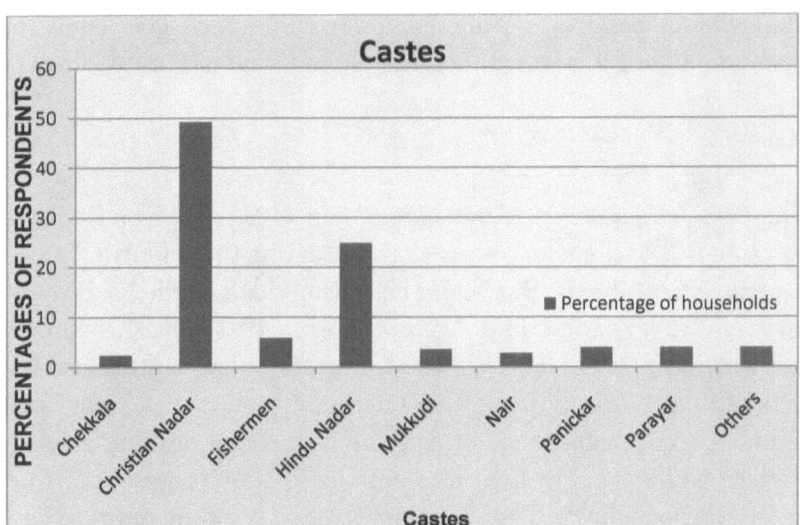

Community

The caste composition does not picture the actual nature of their social status. Hence households belonging to different castes are classified according to their respective communities. The sample households are treated equal on the basis of communities in getting various welfare oriented benefits of the Governments. The distribution of households according to their respective communities is furnished in Table 6.7.

Table 6.7: Community

Community	Frequency	Percentage
Scheduled Caste	20	7.8
Scheduled Tribe	2	0.8
Most Backward Class	8	3.1
Backward Class	199	77.1
Others	29	11.2
Total	258	100.0

It is evident that a substantial share (77.1 percent) of the Chikungunya affected sample households hails from Backward Classes. Since the district has fewer shares of Scheduled Castes and Scheduled Tribes, the sample representations of these communities represent 7.8 and 0.8 percentages respectively. Others are the forward caste households who stand a distant second place with 11.2 percent share.

Figure 6.3: Communities of households

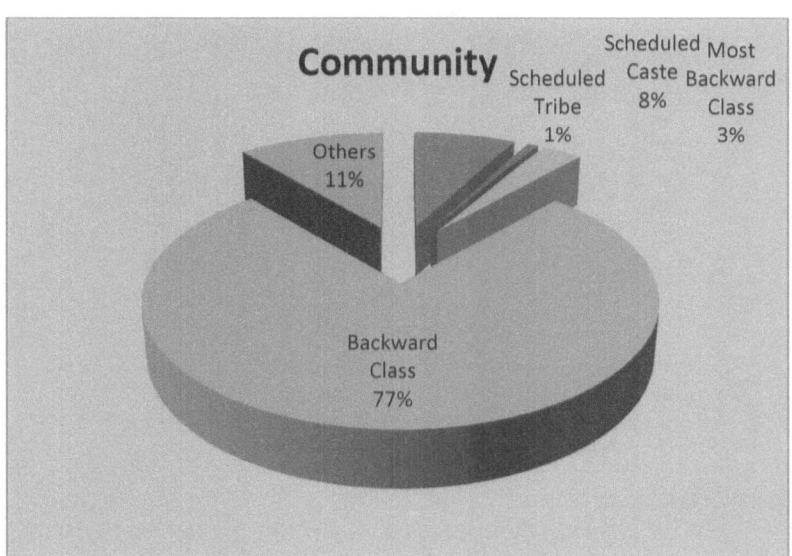

Religion

The distribution of households according to their religion is shown in Table 6.8.

Table 6.8: Religion

Religion	Frequency	Percentage
Hindu	100	38.8
Christian	156	60.5
Muslim	1	0.4
Others	1	0.4
Total	258	100.0

It is found that three – fifth of the sample households (60.5 percent) are Christians. Hindus represent 38.8 percent. The presence of Muslim and other religions comprises only 0.4 percent each respectively.

Figure 6.4: Religious composition of households

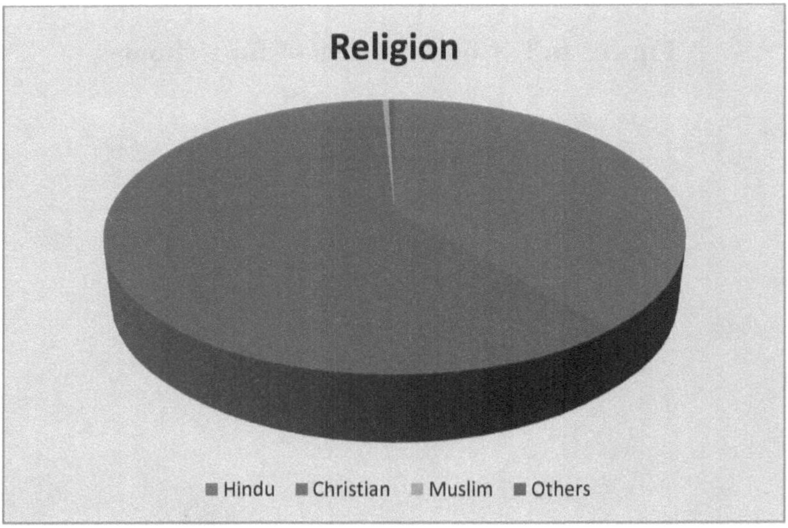

Mother Tongue

The mother tongue of the sample households is shown in Table 6.9.

Table 6.9: Mother tongue

Mother Tongue	Frequency	Percentage
Tamil	216	83.7
Malayalam	42	16.3
Total	258	100.0

Four out of every five households (83.7 percent) are Tamil speaking. The rest (16.3 percent) converses in Malayalam. No other language is found among the sample households.

Type of Family

The type of family of the sample households is shown in Table 6.10.

Table 6.10: Type of family

Type of Family	Frequency	Percentage
Nuclear	223	86.4
Joint	31	12.0
Uni-member	4	1.6
Total	258	100.0

The culture and literacy of the households are found similar in both urban and rural areas. The urban culture supports and instrumental for the division of families into nuclear households. Out of the 258 households 86.4 percent are nuclear. The nuclear family is a family having only one married couple and a common cooking arrangement. It is interesting to note that 1.6 percent of the households are uni-member households. The remaining 12 percent of the households are joint families. Most of the households are nuclear, since the parents also live in nearby residences, somehow maintaining the usual bonds of members as we find in joint families.

Figure 6.5: Type of family (in percentage)

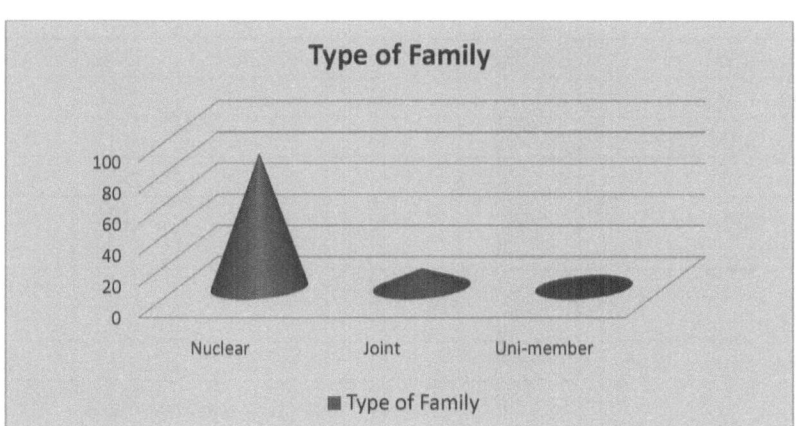

Household Demographic Composition

A household comprises members belonging to different age groups and sex. Age-wise classification of a household is broadly classified into children, working aged population and aged population. The health care needs, health problems and economic impact are not the same for all these age groups. Moreover the health problems and their causes are different for women from that of men.

The details of the household composition are shown in Table 6.11.

The average size of the household is 3.9 with 1.91 male and 1.90 female members. It is found that 98.1 of the households have male members as compared to 99.6 percent of the households having female members. Only 34.9 percent (90 out of 258) of the households have members below 15 years of age. Those households comprise 1.27 male members and 1.24 female members representing 70 and 58 households respectively. It is interesting to note that 98 percent of the average number of households with children have school going children. Thus the demographic structure of the households shows healthy demographic composition of any developed Sate.

Table 6.11: Descriptive statistics of household composition

Variables	Number	Minimum	Maximum	Mean	Standard Deviation
Household size	258	1.00	8.00	3.864	1.254
Male members	253	1.00	5.00	1.905	0.929
Female members	257	1.00	5.00	1.903	0.867
Male Children	70	1.00	3.00	1.271	0.479
Female children	58	1.00	3.00	1.241	0.470
children	90	1.00	3.00	1.656	0.603
School-going male children	61	1.00	3.00	1.246	0.471
School-going female children	52	1.00	3.00	1.250	0.479
School-going children	87	1.00	3.00	1.621	0.595

Activity Status of Household Composition

The working aged population is the active population aged between above 14 and below 60 years of age. Those aged 60 years and above are called the aged population. But there are unemployed persons in the working age and employed people among the aged.

The descriptive statistics of the activity status of the household population is shown in Table 6.12.

It is evident that 2.9 members of an average household size of 3.9 are in the working age group of 15 to 59 years. The average size of the female members in the working age (1.63) appears slightly bigger than that of the same of male members (1.55). It is found those 93 percent (240 out of 258) households have working aged members. However, households with employed male members are almost four times that of the same of households with employed female members.

Table 6.12: Descriptive statistics of employment

Variable	Number	Minimum	Maximum	Mean	Standard Deviation
Working aged men	236	1.00	4.00	1.547	0.816
Working aged women	237	1.00	5.00	1.603	0.830
Total working aged	240	1.00	7.00	2.892	1.327
Employed men	232	1.00	4.00	1.297	0.691
Employed women	64	1.00	4.00	1.312	0.687
Total employed	241	1.00	8.00	1.539	1.040
Aged male workers	43	1.00	1.00	1.000	0.000
Aged female workers	25	1.00	1.00	1.000	0.000
Total aged workers	51	1.00	2.00	1.314	0.469

The average male members employed are 1.30 as compared to 1.31 of the average female members employed. It is found from the survey that households with aged workers account for 19.8 percent (51out of 258). More households have aged male employed members when compared to aged female employed members.

Illiteracy and Marital Status

The descriptive statistics of illiteracy and marital status of household members is shown in Table 6.13.

It is found that 23.26 percent (60 out of 258) of the households have illiterate members. The male illiterate members are found in less numbers (12.4 percent) when compared to the number of households with female illiterate members (20.16 percent). However, it is important that no household has more than one male or female illiterate member.

Table 6.13: Descriptive statistics of illiteracy and marital status

Variable	Households	Minimum	Maximum	Mean	Standard Deviation
Illiterate male	32	1.00	1.00	1.000	0.000
Illiterate female	52	1.00	1.00	1.000	0.000
Total illiterates	60	1.00	2.00	1.417	0.497
Married male	239	1.00	3.00	1.088	0.325
Married female	248	1.00	3.00	1.125	0.377
Total married	250	1.00	12.00	2.176	0.923

The average illiterate members are calculated as 1.42 in 60 households. The data reveals that the average married in the household is 2.18. The average size of female married members is 1.13 as compared to 1.11 of male married members.

Economic Characteristics

Economic characteristics of the households are broadly classified into household income, household expenditure, household savings, household indebtedness and household wealth.

Monthly Household Income

The sample households generate income through various sources. On the whole, the respondent is the main bread winner of the family who is supported by other earning members. Households receive income from other sources such as yield from agriculture, transfer earnings etc. The descriptive statistics of monthly income of the sample households is shown in Table 6.14.

Table 6.14: Descriptive statistics of household income

Variable	Number	Minimum	Maximum	Mean	Standard Deviation
Male income earners (No)	239	1.00	4.00	1.293	0.672
Female income earners (No)	62	1.00	2.00	1.097	0.298
Income earners(No)	250	1.00	5.00	1.512	0.846
Income of the respondent (Mtly)	238	1000.00	80000.00	6974.16	7969.794
Income of family members(Mtly)	93	200.00	85000.00	8932.26	12822.45
Income from other sources(Mtly)	203	250.00	40000.00	2853.20	4099.043
Monthly average household income	258	1000.00	160000.0	12264.5	15611.79

It is interesting to note that 8 households (3.1 percent) do not earn any income through employment to support their family. The survey revealed that those respondents either use the money earned by other members in the family or they receive income from other sources. Out of the 258 households, 92.25 percent have at least one male income earner when compared to 24.03 of the households with at least one female earner. Moreover maximum number of male income earner in a household is 4 when compared to 2 in the case of the female income earning households. Though the average income of the respondents (Rs. 6974.16) shows lesser amount when compared to other family members, (Rs. 8932.26) the latter is the collective contribution ranging from single earner to the maximum of four. Another important point is that three out of every four households (78.68 percent or 203 out 258 households) receive a monthly income of Rs.2853 from other sources. On an average, a household in the study area earn a monthly income of Rs.12, 264.54. The frequency distribution of monthly household income is shown in Table 6.15.

Table 6.15: Total monthly household income

Monthly Income (in Rs)	Frequency	Percentage
Below 2500	9	3.5
2500 - 5000	54	24.4
5000 - 7500	59	22.9
7500 - 10000	47	18.2
10000 - 12500	13	5.0
12500 - 15000	23	8.9
15000 - 17500	12	4.7
Above 17500	41	15.9
Total	258	100.0

Though the average income appears high it is found that 50.8 percent or half of the total sample households earn a monthly income of less than Rs. 7500. Thereafter in every higher income class the frequency shows a continuous decline till the highest income class, however, the highest monthly income class of Rs.17500 and above represents 15.9 percent of the total numbers of households. The distribution of household income reveals that Chikungunya fever is not the disease of the poor households. Many higher income households are also become the victims of the infectious disease.

Figure 6.6: Household monthly income

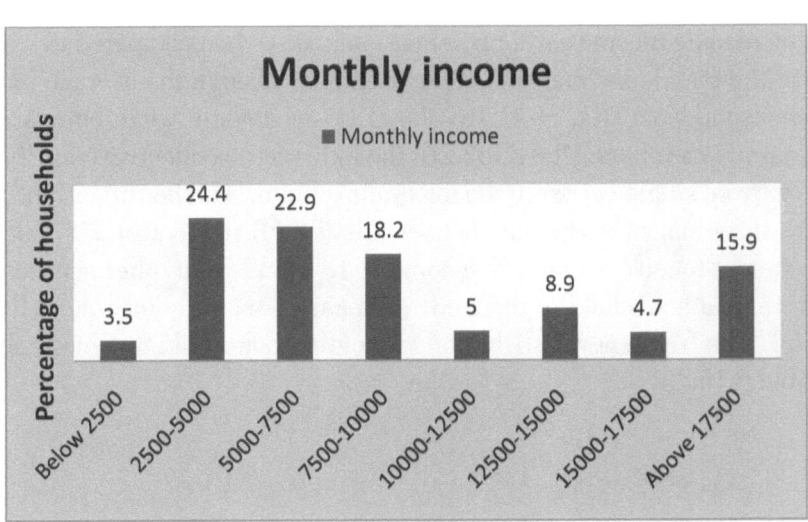

Monthly Household Expenditure

Monthly household expenditure is also another indicator of economic status of a household like monthly household income. A household purchases goods and services on a daily, weekly, monthly, and annual or for a longer term basis. However, all the expenditure made by a household in a year is transformed on a monthly basis. The descriptive statistics of household average monthly expenditure on food items is presented in Table 6.16.

Table 6.16: Monthly expenditure on food

Expenditure mode	Number	Minimum (in Rs)	Maximum (in Rs)	Mean (in Rs)	Standard Deviation
Food taken outside home	228	50.0	6000.0	526.91	532.28
Food prepared at home	258	800.0	9000.0	2347.67	940.77
Total expenditure on food	258	200.0	15000.0	2838.45	1390.49

Food is the only expenditure item referred to the entire sample households. For the purpose of estimating expenditure on both foods taken outside home and at home were taken into account. Among the total sample households, 88.37 percent (228) have incurred an expenditure on food taken outside their home. The monthly average expenditure on food taken outside home is estimated as Rs.526.91. All the sample households incurred expenditure for the preparation of food at home. The average monthly expenditure on food is Rs.2838.45 which is 23.14 percent of their average monthly household income. The descriptive statistics of different household consumption items is shown in Table 6.17.

It is surprising to note that debt repayment inclusive of the principal and interest occupies the second largest expenditure item after food even though only 158 of the 258 households are indebted. The next important item of expenditure is the expenditure on education of Rs.679.22. The priorities of households on various items of expenditure not only show their socio- economic condition; but also their expenditure pattern based on their cultural background.

Figure 6.7: Average monthly household expenditure

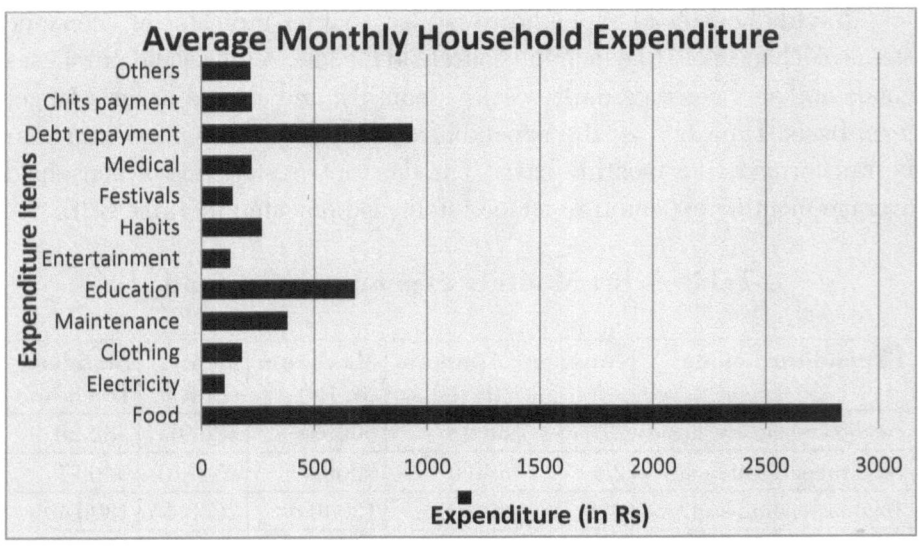

Table 6.17: Descriptive statistics of household expenditure items

Expenditure Items	Households	Minimum	Maximum	Mean	Standard Deviation
Food	258	200.00	15000.00	2835.930	1391.602
Electricity	248	15.00	1047.00	103.4516	89.076
Clothing	255	20.00	2500.00	179.6588	235.334
Maintenance	184	10.00	6000.00	380.6250	843.005
Education	144	15.00	15000.00	679.2153	1507.217
Entertainment	234	50.00	1000.00	129.7863	69.083
Habits	178	5.00	3900.00	267.9494	349.600
Festivals	254	25.00	750.00	139.3583	103.760
Medical	245	15.00	4000.00	221.9796	365.182
Debt repayment	158	50.00	5000.00	936.3924	837.171
Chits payment	170	3.00	2000.00	224.1588	332.729
Others	177	25.00	1200.00	218.5311	144.803
Total	258	1080.00	40000.00	5487.763	3561.858

Table 6.18 shows the frequency the distribution of average monthly household expenditure of the sample households.

Table 6.18: Total average monthly household expenditure

Monthly Household Expenditure (in Rs.)	Frequency	Percentage
Below 2000	5	1.9
2001 -4000	78	30.2
4001 -6000	110	42.6
6001 -8000	32	12.4
Above 8000	33	12.8
Total	258	100.0

More than two- fifth of the sample households (42.6 percent) incur expenditure between Rs. 4000 and Rs.6000 per month. Households belong to the monthly expenditure of less than Rs.4000 account for 32.1 percent. The monthly household expenditure classes of Rs.6000 -8000 and above Rs.8000 have a percent share of 12.4 and 12.8 respectively. The average monthly household expenditure is estimated as Rs. 5487.76 with a standard deviation of 3561.86.

Household Saving

The particulars of household saving are shown in Table 6.19.

Table 6.19: Saving households

Savings	Households	Percentage
Yes	145	56.2
No	113	43.8
Total	258	100.0

Out of 258 household 56.2 percent affirmed possessing some amount as savings at the time of survey. It is reported during the survey that all those having savings are in some commercial banks and others are in chits. Most of the women having savings are members in self help groups. Chits are common among male members. The household average savings is estimated as Rs. 17976 with a standard deviation of 44991.26.The frequency distribution of household savings is presented in Table 6.20.

It is evident from the data that nearly one third (33.1 percent) of those household have savings is in the lowest class of less than Rs. 3000, however 20 percent of the households having savings represent in the highest savings group of Rs.18000 and above. Similarly the same representation of 20 percent is recorded in the second lowest saving class of Rs.3000 Rs.6000.

Table 6.20: Present household savings

Savings (in Rs.)	Frequency	Percentage
Below 3000	48	33.1
3001 - 6000	29	20.0
6001 - 9000	17	11.7
9000 - 12000	16	11.0
12000 - 15000	4	2.8
15001 - 18000	2	1.4
Above 18000	29	20.0
Total	145	100.0

These three groups collectively constitute 73.1 percent or almost three fourth of the households with savings. The remaining 27.9 percent households have savings ranged between Rs.6000 Rs.18000.

Household Debt

The details of households indebted are shown in Table 6.21.

Table 6.21: Indebted households

Indebtedness	Households	Percentage
Yes	184	71.3
No	74	28.7
Total	258	100.0

It is surprised to note that 71.3 percent of the sample households are debtors. It is observed that they mainly borrowed money for construction, education and marriage purposes. Small debts are mainly for consumption and medical purposes. The frequency distribution of households according to the level of indebtedness is shown Table 6.22.

Table 6.22: Level of household indebtedness

Level of household indebtedness (in Rs.)	Frequency	Percentage
Below - 25000	49	26.6
25001 - 50000	53	28.8
50001 - 75000	14	7.6
75001 - 100000	25	13.6
100001 - 125000	7	3.8
125001 - 150000	8	4.3
175001 - 200000	12	6.5
Above - 200000	16	8.7
Total	184	100.0

Households in the lowest indebtedness classes between Rs.25000 and Rs.50000 account for 28.8 percent. More than half (55.4 percent) of the indebted households represent the lowest two classes of the level of household indebtedness. Households representing the highest debt class of Rs. 2 lakhs and above accounting for 8.7 percent. The third ranking debt class is Rs.75001-100000 accounting for 13.6 percent of the indebted households. The average household debt is computed as Rs.102958.42 with a standard deviation of 44991.26. It is clear that indebtedness is deep-rooted among the sample households and the intensity of debt is also very high.

Household Wealth

The household's wealth is an assessment of the value of landed properties inclusive of house and other valuable items possessed by the household. The frequency distribution of households according to their levels of wealth is shown in Table 6.23.

Discussions with the respondents revealed that land is the richest possession of the households besides their houses and Jewels. The wealth of households includes both land and other properties. In addition to this, they rear household animals such as cattle and poultry.

Figure 6.8: Average level of household indebtedness

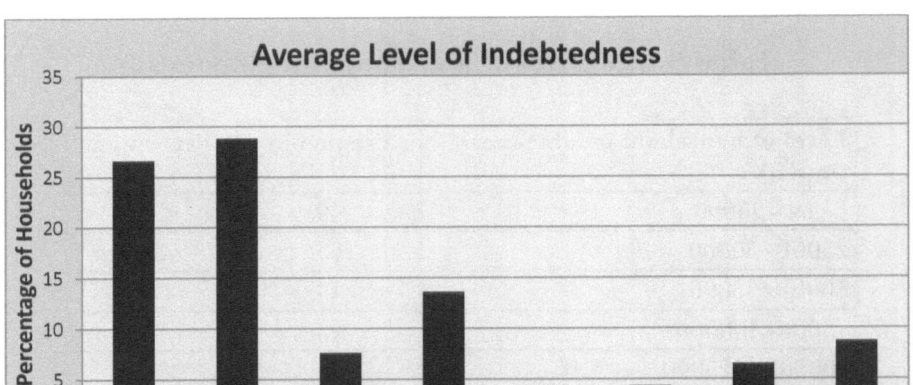

Table 6.23: Levels of household wealth (in Rs. lakhs)

Levels of household wealth	Frequency	Percentage
Below 2	37	14.3
2 -- 4	72	27.9
4 -- 6	45	17.4
6 – 8	29	11.2
8 – 10	24	9.3
10 – 12	3	1.2
12 -- 14	2	.8
14 and Above	46	17.8
Total	258	100.0

The frequency distribution of sample households according to their levels of wealth shows that more than one fourth (27.9 percent) of the households possess wealth valued between Rs.200000 and Rs.400000. Only 14.3 percent of the households have wealth less than 2 lakhs. However, 17. 8 percent of the household are found in the highest wealth class of Rs.14 lakhs and above. The average possession of assets by the households is valued at Rs. 8.27 lakhs with a standard deviation of 1003182.34.

Figure 6.9: Household wealth

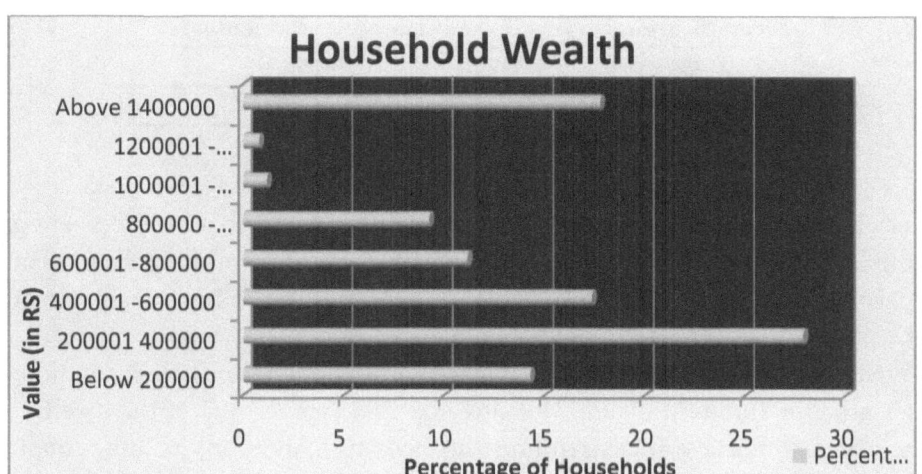

Housing

Housing details of the sample households outline their living environment. The nature of residency of the sample households is given in Table 6.24.

Table 6.24: Nature of tenancy

Nature of tenancy	Frequency	Percentage
Owned	253	98.1
Rented	5	1.9
Total	258	100.0

It is evident that almost all the sample households own their residence, except an insignificant proportion of 1.9 percent. Tenants are mostly people who come from distant places for work or people who have lost their houses due to some economic reasons or accident.

Table 6.25 shows electrifications of the residences.

Table 6.25: Electrification of house

Electrification	Frequency	Percentage
Yes	248	96.1
No	10	3.9
Total	258	100.0

Electrified houses adds amenity to life. It is found that 96.1 percent of the 258 houses are electrified. Un-electrified houses are the interior semi permanent habitations with thatched roof. Most of these houses are owned by people from the poor socio economic sections of the society.

Ownership and electrification are necessary but not sufficient condition for a better standard of life. Housing size and type of roof of the dwelling are also important in explaining the housing conditions of the sample households. Hence the housing area of the houses of the respondents are approximately assessed and presented in Table 6.26.

Table 6.26: Housing area

Housing area (in sq.ft)			Frequency	Percentage
Below 500			61	23.6
501 - 750			87	33.7
751 - 1000			82	31.8
Above 1000			28	10.9
Total			258	100.0
	N	Minimum	Maximum	Mean	Std. Deviation
Area	258	100.0	2400.00	748.74	320.520

In general, the size of area occupied for housing purpose is adequate. Less than one fourth (23.6 percent) of the sample households lived in houses of less than 500 sq.ft. Households representing the housing area class of 501 -750 sq.ft are the largest accounting for 33.7 percent. Housing area of 751–1000 sq.ft represents 31.8 percent of the households. Houses above 1000 sq.ft account for 10.9 percent of the sample households. The average housing area of the sample households is 748.74 sq.ft. with a standard deviation of 320.52.

Figure 6.10: Area of house

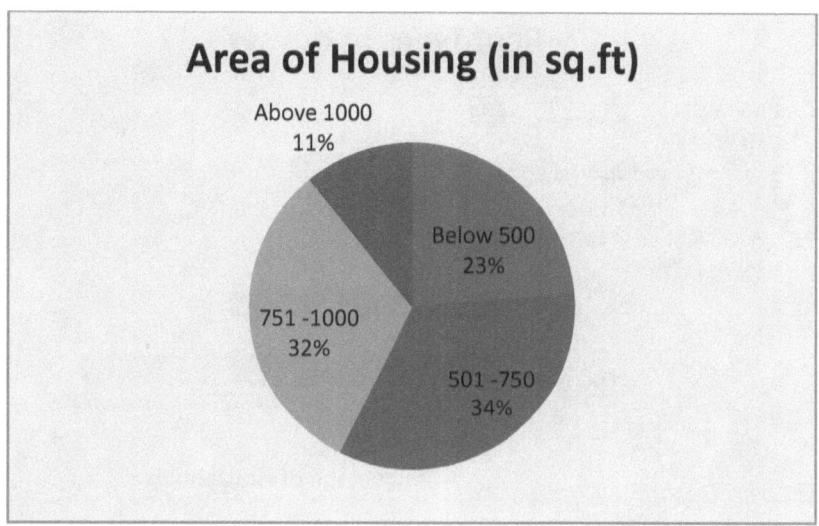

Nature of the house-roof is another important indicator of housing environment. The frequency distribution of households having different types of roof in their building is presented in Table 6.27.

Table 6.27: Nature of roof of house

Nature of roof	Households	Percentage
Concrete	144	55.8
Tiled	92	35.7
Roof made up of coconut leaves	10	3.9
Roof made up of hay/ straws	2	.8
others	10	3.9
Total	258	100.0

It is interesting to note that more than half (55.8 percent) of the households possesses houses with concrete roof. The next biggest share of 35.7 percent of the households has houses with tiled roof. Roofs made-up of coconut leaves and roof of hay and straw account for 3.9 and 0.8 percentages respectively.

Figure 6.11: Roof types of houses

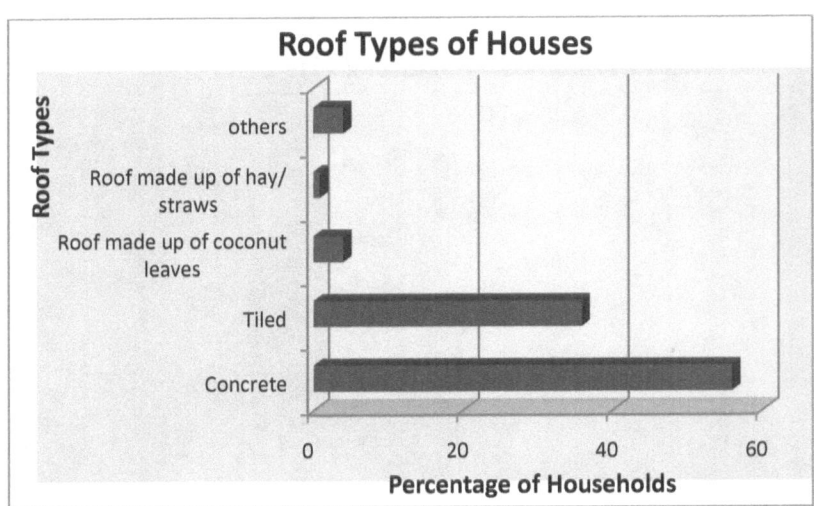

The descriptive statistics of the number of windows and number of rooms of the houses of sample households is shown in Table 6.28.

Table 6.28: Descriptive statistics of windows and rooms

Variables	N	Minimum	Maximum	Mean	Std. Deviation
Number of windows	258	1.00	13.00	5.135	2.261
Number of rooms	258	1.00	8.00	3.166	1.206

The average number of windows and rooms are worked out as 5.14 and 3.2 with a standard deviation of 2.261 and 1.206 respectively.

The frequency distribution of houses with numbers of windows is shown in Table 6.29.

Table 6.29: Number of windows

Number of windows	Frequency	Percentage
One	2	.8
Two	27	10.5
Three	36	14.0
Four	49	19.0

Five	39	15.1
Six	44	17.1
Seven	21	8.1
Eight	24	9.3
Nine	5	1.9
Ten	6	2.3
More than ten	5	2.0
Total	258	100.0

It is clear that single window- houses form 0.8 percent of the houses. Maximum houses (19.0 percent) have four windows. Houses having less than four windows account for 25.3 percent and houses with more than four windows comprise 55.8 percent of the total houses of the respondents. This clearly indicates that most of the houses have proper ventilation and have enough space.

Table 6.30 shows the distribution of houses according to number of rooms.

Table 6.30: Number of rooms

Number of rooms	Frequency	Percentage
One	9	3.5
Two	72	27.9
Three	91	35.3
Four	55	21.3
Five	21	8.1
Six	5	1.9
Seven	4	1.6
Eight	1	0.4
Total	258	100.0

More than one-third of the houses (35.3 percent) have three rooms. Houses with two rooms account for 27.9 percent. Houses with four, five and six rooms account for 21.3, 8.1 and 1.9 percentages respectively of the total houses. Hence if number of windows and rooms are taken as the indices of better housing facilities, majority of the houses have adequate ventilation and living space.

Access Way to Residence

Access way to the house plays an important part in explaining the possibility of providing immediate medical attention in case of any medical emergency to the members of the households. The different types of access ways to the houses of the sample households is shown in Table 6.31.

Vehicular road is the access way to the residences of 47.3 percent of the sample households. However, paved path and unpaved path are not suitable for vehicular transport which account for 42.6 and 9.3 percentages respectively of the total households.

Table 6.31: Access way to the house

Access way to house	Frequency	Percentage
Vehicular road	122	47.3
Paved path	110	42.6
Unpaved path	24	9.3
Others	2	0.8
Total	258	100.0

Unpaved path is difficult to travel and such places are found in interior areas. In general, road network is satisfactory in the selected areas of the study.

Table 6.32 gives the distance between residence and the vehicular road of the sample households.

Table 6.32: Distance between residence and vehicular road

Distance (in metres)	Frequency	Percentage
Below 200	146	56.6
200 -400	18	7.0
400 -600	28	10.9
600 -800	11	4.3
800 -1000	32	12.4
1000 -1200	2	.8

1200 -1400			1	.4	
Above1400			20	7.8	
Total			258	100.0	
	N	Minimum	Maximum	Mean	Std. Deviation
Distance	258	5.00	6000.00	495.077	836.328

It is interesting to note that 46.9 percent of the residences are located 200 metres away from the vehicular road. Residences above 1400 metres from the vehicular road account for 7.8 percent. In these households members have to travel difficult terrains to reach the vehicular road. The second and third largest numbers of households are found in the distance classes of 800-1000 and 400-600 metres between residence and vehicular road. The average distance between residence and vehicular road is estimated 495.08 metres with a standard decoration of 836.33.

Figure 6.12: Distance between residence and vehicular road

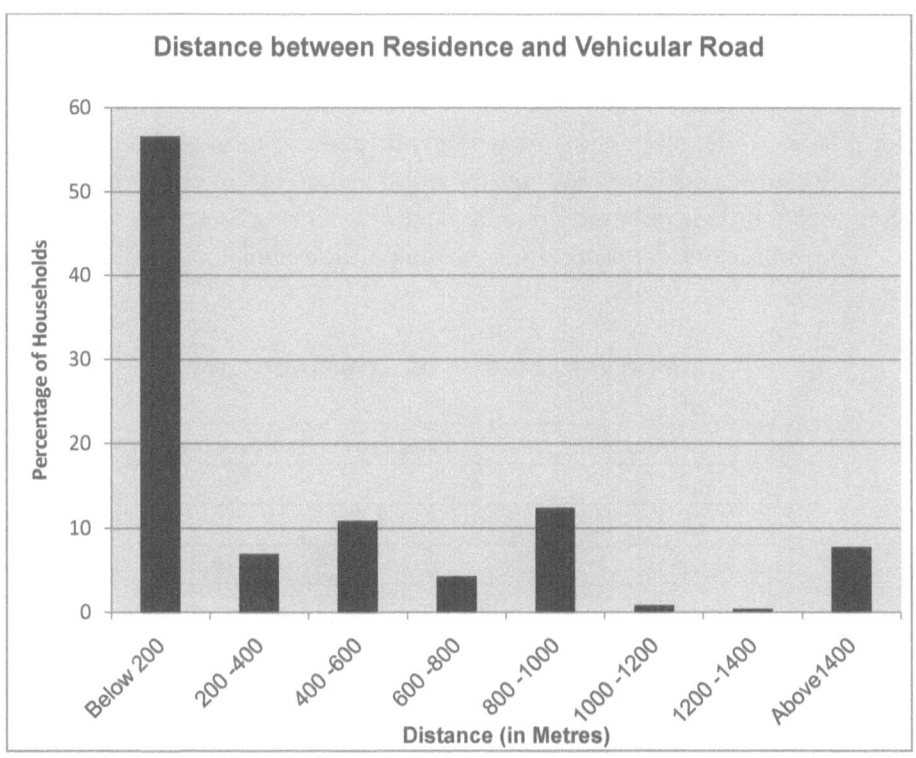

Residential Environment

The quality of residential environment is important for protecting people from the infection of communicable diseases. Water stagnating area, drinking water source, water storage, waste disposal, presence of open area, residence near banana and rubber plantations, toilets and rearing of cattle and pet animals are indentified as the variables related to residential environment.

Table 6.33 shows the presence of water stagnating areas near the residences of the sample households.

Table 6.33: Presence of water stagnating area

Water stagnating area	Frequency	Percentage
Yes	128	49.6
No	130	50.4
Total	258	100.0

Nearly half (49.6 percent) of the residences are located near water stagnating areas. Water stagnation is one of the important causes for breeding mosquitoes. The topography of the study area is with ups and down hence water stagnating areas are with water in most of the times in a year. Moreover residences are mostly found isolated from others hence the open areas in their proximity provide opportunities for water stagnation.

The sources of drinking water of sample households are presented in Table 6.34.

Table 6.34: Source of drinking water

Source	Frequency	Percentage
Open well	121	46.9
Bore well	33	12.8
Public tap	104	40.3
Total	258	100.0

Three important sources of drinking water in the selected area are openwell, public tap and bore well. Open well is the main source for drinking water and it accounts for 46.9 percent of the sample households. Each house has an open well within the compound wall if it is an independent house. Tap water is the source of drinking water for those who reside close to the pavements and vehicular roads. Households depending on public tap for drinking purpose account for 40.3 percent. Bore well is a source of drinking water in the localities of town where open space close to their residence is less. Bore well as a source of drinking water accounts for 12.8 percent of the households.

Households store water in different types of containers. They include overhead tank, pots and open storage tank. The details of water storing mechanism of the sample households are furnished in Table 6.35.

Table 6.35: Water storage

Type of water storage	Frequency	Percentage
Overhead tank	113	43.8
Pots	123	47.7
Open storage tank	21	8.1
Others	1	.4
Total	258	100.0

Pots and overhead tank are the two common water storing methods adopted by the households. These two methods of water storing are adopted by 47.7 and 43.8 percentages respectively of the sample households. Open storages and other methods comprise very insignificant share of 8.1 and 0.4 percentages of the households. Observations in the study area revealed that drinking water storage is a less important cause of mosquito breeding because most of the overhead tanks and the pots remain closed in most of the households.

Waste disposal appears to be one of the important reasons for the growth of mosquito. The areas of waste disposal of the sample households are shown in Table 6.36.

Table 6.36: Waste disposal area

Area of waste disposal	Frequency	Percentage
In the backyard	115	44.6
In the disposal site	116	45.0
Burn it for cooking	27	10.5
Total	258	100.0

It is found that 44.6 percent of the households dispose waste in their backyards. The biodegradable waste gradually disappears by natural decomposition because land area available in the backyard is comparatively large for decomposition. However, coconut shell, cycle tire, unused or broken pots, plastic containers etc do not decompose in short duration hence store water during the monsoon season. In such households the Chik mosquitoes breed in pure water in the monsoon season. Many of the households replied that they use coconut shell mostly as a cooking fuel because they are relatively better efficient fuel when compared to other bio-fuels. Disposal site was the disposal area for 44.6 percent of the households. However, site inspection revealed that disposal site they mean is a place for the disposal of waste. Such wastes are not cleared from these sites in majority of the cases, except in a few places where houses are located in municipal areas. It is interesting to note that 10.5 percent of the households use waste as cooking fuel or as organic manure for banana trees and vegetables. In these houses also non-biodegradable wastes are thrown in open.

Presence of open area near house may be used for waste disposal in many of the sample households. Ditches in open areas also store water during the rainy season. Table 6.37 classifies households on the basis of having open area, banana plantation and rubber plantation near their residences.

Table 6.37: Presence of various mosquito breeding facilities near house

Mosquito breeding facilities	Households	Percentage
Open area	135	52.3
Banana plantations	181	70.2
Rubber plantations	159	61.6

More than half (52.3 percent) of the sample households have open area near their house. It is important to note that 70.2 percent of the households have banana plantations and 61.6 percent of the households have rubber plantations near their house. Banana plantations and rubber plantations are the places where water store during monsoon. Banana plantations have water storing pit lanes where water stagnates during rainy season. In rubber plantations coconut shell is used for collecting tapped rubber. After collecting rubber, the empty shells store water in rainy seasons. These are suspected as the two important reasons for water storing resulting the breeding of Aedes mosquitoes.

Table 6.38 shows availability of toilet facilities for the sample households.

Table 6.38: Toilet facility

Toilet facility	Frequency	Percentage
Yes	177	68.6
No	81	31.4
Total	258	100.0

The survey showed that people in the study area have better health consciousness. More than two-thirds (68.6 percent) of the people have separate closed toilet facilities attached to their house. Only 31.4 percent defecate in open places, such households are found in the interior areas.

Rearing of cattle and pet animals degrade the living environment. Households rearing cattle or pet animals are shown in Table 6.39.

Table 6.39: Rearing of cattle / pet animals

Cattle/ pet animals	Frequency	Percentage
Yes	71	27.5
No	187	72.5
Total	258	100.0

More than one-fourth (27.5 percent) of the total sample households rear cattle or pet animals. Cattle rearing are not found in three-fourth of the households. Hence the available evidences justify that banana plantations, rubber plantations and open area with bush and pits are the basic reasons for the meridian growth of mosquitoes in the study areas during monsoons.

Since Chikungunya fever is caused by environmental influences, most of the infections are involuntary. It inflicts problem to all sections of people at all ages but it is vulnerable to people in poor environment and people in the poor socio economic strata of the society. The disease is less among female children but among the working aged population, females are the worst affected. The occurrence of the disease among the aged is deplorable because of their less immune condition and the prevalence of other common diseases pertinent to the old people.

Health Conditions And The Extent Of Illness In Chikungunya Affected Households In Kanyakumari District

ealth conditions and the extent of illness of Chikungunya fever affected households are examined based on the information obtained from their memory of illness episode. The information collected from the households in the study area is with respect to the condition of persons affected by Chikungunya fever during 2007. The details comprise the gender composition of the sick persons, their age, and work force participation, history of health effects, treatment, the impact of illness on employment and the total cost of illness at the household level. In particular the present chapter studies the intensity of the disease at the household level, various symptoms of the disease to the sick persons with special significance and the estimation of cost of illness due to Chikungunya fever.

Health is a balance between the physical and social environment and infection of Chikungunya fever can disturb the balance and strike the livelihood in different ways. Difference in symptoms and economic and social inabilities to a delayed diagnosis potentially encourage the households to incur more expenditure than what is actually required. Chikungunya fever is a non-fatal disease and the general medical prescription is rest, more water intake and if necessary the intake of mild pain killer. But evidences show that it played havoc in the region, causing uncertainty and medical emergency. Severity, symptoms and hardships of the disease differ between groups of people from differing socio- economic strata. Treating a sense of seriousness to the disease makes the households demand treatment at a higher price. The conditions of the affected people after the recovery from fever make further suspicions about the disease. Many of them feel all the health problems are due to the infection of Chikungunya. The general objective of treating a disease is for the recovery of the patient; however Chikungunya fever has made prolonged health impairment to many of the victims even after their recovery of the fever in different forms. Its

economic impact on the household is similar to a trauma. The present
chapter describes the health conditions of Chikungunya affected households
in the Kanyakumari district of Tamil Nadu.

Intensity of Chikungunya Fever

Chikungunya fever is an epidemic affected to a large number of
households in monsoon season in many years in succession since 2006.
The household survey conducted for the present study is on those
households where members affected by Chikungunya fever in 2007 and
the subsequent cost of illness to the household. The basics of the infection
of the disease on the members are different. It affected different age groups
and sexes indiscriminately. Table 7.1 shows the descriptive statistics of the
Chikungunya affected sample households in Kanyakumari District.

The average number of members affected by Chikungunya fever is 1.56
having a minimum of one and a maximum of 5 persons in a household with a
standard deviation of 0.826. It is found that only 7.36 percent (19 out of 258)
of the sample households have children affected by Chikungunya fever as
compared to 7.36 percent of households with male children and 4.26 percent
(11 out of 258) households with female children. Not only children are less
affected in general but female children are less affected than male children.
The average number of male children affected is 1.1 as compared to 1.0 of
female children. Most of the children remain in the house for most of the time
in a day and the infection may be mostly from the mosquito outside home.

Table 7.1: Descriptive statistics of
Chikungunya affected households

Category of people affected	N	Minimum	Maximum	Mean	Std. Deviation
Total members	258	1.00	5.00	1.5620	.8263
Male children	19	1.00	2.00	1.1053	.3153
Female children	11	1.00	1.00	1.0000	.0000
Total children	19	1.00	2.00	1.2632	.4524
Working age male population	142	1.00	3.00	1.0704	.2830
Working age female population	170	1.00	3.00	1.1353	.3913
Total working age population	222	1.00	4.00	1.4685	.7222
Aged members	42	1.00	2.00	1.2857	.4572

The members affected in the working age group comprise 86.05 percent (222 out 258) of the sample households. Unlike children, in the working age group, more households (65.89 percent or 170 out of 258) had women members affected by Chikungunya than households with male members (55.04 percent or 142 out of 258). The average number of female members affected is 1.4 as compared to 1.07 of male members. Households having aged members affected by the fever are 16.28 percent (42 out of 258) showing an average of 1.29 members. The average figure shows that more members in the working age are affected followed by aged members and children.

The average figures do not give a clear picture about the intensity of the disease on different households. Hence the households are distributed according to the number of members affected. The details are furnished in Table 7.2.

It is found that more than three- fifth (61.2 percent) of the households have a single member in their family affected by Chikungunya fever in the reference year.

Table 7.2: Number of members affected by Chikungunya

Number of members affected	Households	Percentage
One	158	61.2
Two	65	25.2
Three	26	10.1
Four	8	3.1
Five	1	.4
Total	258	100.0

Two- members affected households form one- fourth (25.2 percent). The general tendency of the frequency distribution is that less number of households is found in the category higher number of household members affected. Households with three, four and five members affected account for 10.1, 3.1 and 0.4 percentages respectively of the total households.

In order to understand the infliction Chikungunya fever based on demography, households having children and working aged population are classified according to sex. Table 7.3 shows the distribution of households on the basis of number of male children and female children affected.

Table 7.3: Number of male children affected

Male children	Households	Percentage
One	17	89.5
Two	2	10.5
Total	19	100.0
Female children		
One	11	100.0

Figure 7.1: Chikungunya affected households

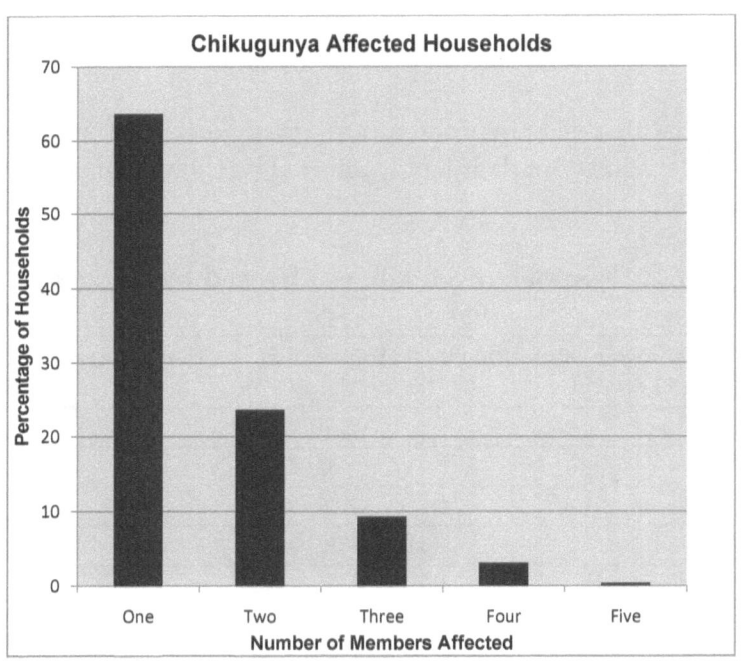

It is clear that 89.5 percent of the male children households have a single male children affected, while the same is 100 percent in the case of households having female children affected. No household has more than one female children affected. The frequency distribution of children affected households is shown in Table 7.4.

Table 7.4: Total children affected

Total children	Households	Percentage
One	14	73.7
Two	5	26.3
Total	19	100.0

Single children affected household forms 73.7 percent of the total children affected households. Two children affected households account for 26.3 percent. No household has more than two children affected. Out of the 258 households only 7.36 percent have children affected by Chikungunya fever showing lesser infection of Chikungunya among children.

Information on working age population affected is given in the form of descriptive statistics. The intensity of Chikungunya fever is indicated by the infection of the disease among number of people in the working age group. Table 7.5 presents the distribution of households according to the number of male members affected in the working age group

Table 7.5: Working age male members affected

Working aged male population	Households	Percentage
One	133	93.7
Two	8	5.6
Three	1	.7
Total	142	100.0

Table 7.5 points out that 93.7 percent of the households having male members affected in the working age group by Chikungunya fever have a single member affected. Households with two and three male members affected represent 5.6 and 0.7 percentages respectively. The distribution of households according to the number of female members affected in the working age group is given in Table 7.6.

Table 7.6: Working age female population affected

Working aged male population	Households	Percentage
One	150	88.2
Two	17	10.0
Three	3	1.8
Total	170	100.0

It is evident that 88.2 percent of the households having women members affected by Chikungunya fever in the working age group reported a single member in this category. Households with two and three female members in the working age category affected accounting for 10 and 1.8 percentages respectively. A comparison of Table 7.5 and 7.6 revealed that not only more number of households has female members in the working age group affected by Chikungunya fever but also more number of female members per household in this age category is affected. And more households are found having women in the working age group than man.

The households are distributed according to the number of members affected in the working age group is shown in Table 7.7.

Table 7.7: Total working age population affected

Working aged population	Frequency	Percentage
One	143	64.4
Two	59	26.6
Three	15	6.8
Four	5	2.3
Total	222	100.0

Households with single member affected in the working age group account for 64.4 percent. More than one – fourth (26.6 percent) of the households reported two members in this category. Only 6.8 and 2.3 percentages respectively of the households have three and four members in the same age group. Since a large number of members in the working age group affected by the Chikungunya fever, it has a direct impact on the household economy. Moreover more number of women members affected made many of the households paralysed. Most of the able bodied men in those households had to act as caretakers during their period of illness.

The frequency distribution of aged members affected is shown in Table 7.8.

Table 7.8: Number of affected aged members

Aged members	Households	Percentage
One	30	71.4
Two	12	28.6
Total	42	100.0

Out of the 42 households having aged members affected by Chikungunya fever 71.4 percent have a single aged member affected. Two aged members affected households share the remaining 28.6 percent.

Nature of Infection

Chikungunya fever is an infected disease cause disability or sickness to one or more than one members in a household. The pattern of infection is not uniform among the different households. In some of the households only a single member is infected while in others all the members affected at a time causing severe hardship to the family in caretaking as well as meeting the means to tackle the hardship. But in some other households it was found that all the members affected but simultaneously by one by one. In other infected households some of its members were affected at a time or simultaneously. The details of the pattern of infection of Chikungunya fever among the sample households is furnished in Table.7.9

Out of the 258 Chikungunya affected households, 63.6 percent reported infection to a single member in their family. The next biggest group comes under the category of some members affected simultaneously. They account for 21.7 percent. All family members affected simultaneously and some members affected in different periods in a year share an equal proportion of 3.9 percent. Only 1.9 percent of the households reported the inflection of Chikungunya fever to all of its members at a time. Since more than three- fifth of the sample households have only one member affected, the hardship faced by these households are manageable. It is really a problem for other households and the degree of hardship depends upon the pattern of infection.

Table 7.9: Nature of infection in the household

Nature of infection	Households	Percentage
All family members affected at a time	5	1.9
All family members affected simultaneously	10	3.9
Some of the members affected at a time	13	5.0
Some of the members affected simultaneously	56	21.7
Some of the members affected in different periods in a year	10	3.9
Only one member affected	164	63.6
Total	258	100.0

Detection

The detection and confirmation of Chikungunya fever is informal. None of the Chikungunya case is on the basis of virology detection conducted by the recognised laboratories. The detection of Chikungunya fever in the selected households is based on clinical examination, clinical symptoms and doctor's diagnosis. Table 7.10 shows the descriptive statistics of households on the basis of the source of detection.

Table 7.10: Descriptive statistics of Chikungunya detection

Source of detection	Households	Minimum	Maximum	Mean	Std. Deviation
Clinical examination	37	1.00	4.00	1.3514	.78938
Clinical symptoms	48	1.00	4.00	1.4792	.74347
Doctor's diagnosis	184	1.00	4.00	1.5000	1.21016

Descriptive statistics reveal that 184 households (71.3 percent) have indentified the fever as Chikungunya after doctor's diagnosis. Some of the households (13.34 percent) claim that they identified Chikungunya after clinical examination. Clinical symptoms were the source of identification for 18.6 percent of the households. It is found that in a single household there were cases with different sources of detection.

Chikungunya fever created panic when people did not have the experience of the fever. Later, clinical symptoms and the common experience of the disease in their proximity helped patients to identify the disease and they confirmed the disease mostly by doctor's diagnosis.

Table 7.11 shows the details of wage earners affected households.

Table 7.11: Wage earners affected

Wage earners affected	Households	Percentage
Yes	167	64.7
No	91	35.3
Total	258	100.0

Majority of the Chikungunya fever affected households (64.7 percent) have at least one wage earner affected by the disease. However, 35.3 percent of the households have children, unemployed members in the working age group or aged members without job affected.

The distribution of households according to the number of wage earners affected is shown in Table 7.12.

Table 7.12: Number of wage earners affected

Wage earners affected	Households	Percentage
One	140	83.8
Two	20	12.0
Three	5	3.0
Four	2	1.2
Total	167	100.0

More than four- fifth (83.8 percent) of the wage earners infected households have a single member affected by the fever. Two, three and four wage earners affected households account for 12, 3 and 1.2 percentages respectively. The pattern of infection shows that the percentages of households affected decline sharply as the number of wage earners affected by the Chikungunya fever increases.

The economic impact of Chikungunya fever is partially explained by the source of medical expense. The details of the source of medical expense are presented in Table 7.13.

Table 7.13: Managing the medical expenses

Managing medical assistance	Households	Percentage
From past savings	97	37.6
Borrowed money	125	48.4
Support from friends and relatives	21	8.1
Depending public health centres	8	3.1
Others	7	2.7
Total	258	100.0

It is reported that nearly half (48.4 percent) of the households borrowed money to meet the medical expenditure for Chikungunya fever. More than one-third (37.6 percent) of the households used their past savings for this purpose. Support from friends and relatives and totally depending on public health services account for 8.1 and 3.1 percentages respectively. Other sources represent only 2.7 percent. Some of the households depend on the public sources for medical facilities; they cannot entirely depend on such sources, however the burden is less for those households.

Chikungunya fever is unforgettable to many of the sick persons. Naturally some of the patients can bear the pain. The extent of the pain suffered by the sick persons on a household basis is assessed. The descriptive statistics is presented in Table 7.14.

Table 7.14: Descriptive statistics of affected persons with varied levels of pain

Levels of pain	Households	Minimum	Maximum	Mean	Std. Deviation
Mild pain	4	1.00	3.00	2.250	.9574
Moderate pain	16	1.00	2.00	1.125	.3415
Severe pain	245	1.00	4.00	1.506	.7976

It is interesting to note that 245 of the total 258 households (94.96 percent) have sick persons circumscribe severe pain. The average sick persons of this category account for 1.5 with a standard deviation of 0.798. The moderate pain cases were reported in 6.2 percent households, while mild pain is the least in only 1.6 percent of the households. Thus it is very clear that the physical pain suffered of the Chikungunya fever is the extreme among the sick persons in almost all households.

Symptoms of Chikungunya Fever

Chikungunya is an infectious disease show varied symptoms based on the age and sex of the sick persons besides the location and season of the inflection. The descriptive statistics of the symptoms of Chikungunya fever is presented in Table 7.15.

Table 7.15: Descriptive statistics of symptoms of Chikungunya fever

Symptoms	Households	Minimum	Maximum	Mean	Std. Deviation
Sudden fever	258	1.00	5.00	1.488	.790
Cough	217	1.00	4.00	1.424	.716
Swelling	178	1.00	3.00	1.365	.588
Chills	129	1.00	4.00	1.333	.629
Headache	216	1.00	4.00	1.407	.668
Nausea	73	1.00	3.00	1.260	.472
Vomiting	150	1.00	4.00	1.360	.678
Joint pain	254	1.00	4.00	1.464	.741
Rash	117	1.00	2.00	1.282	.451
Abdominal pain	190	1.00	4.00	1.310	.636

It is evident that among the symptoms, sudden fever is the only symptom present in sick persons in all the households at the time of its infection. Joint pain is the second most important symptom reported by 98.45 percent of the households. Cough and headache are the third and fourth significant symptoms accounting for 84.11 and 83.72 percentages (217 and 216) respectively of the total households. Fever, cough and headache are the most common symptoms besides joint pain. Joint pain generally is a peculiar feature of backward bending posture which is taken as one of the clinical identifications of Chikungunya fever. Rash and swelling are the special features of Chikungunya fever. These two symptoms are reported by 43.35 percent (117 out of 258) and 68.99 percent (178 out of 258) respectively of the total households. Other important symptoms in the descending order of importance are vomiting, chills and nausea in the percentage of 58.14, 50.0 and 28.29 respectively.

Among these symptoms, joint pain and swelling continued for longer duration, while cough, chills and headache disappear when patient recovers from the fever. The sick persons suffer from the after effects of the fever for a longer time. The details of the households with after effects from Chikungunya fever are shown in Table 7.16.

Table 7.16: After-effects of Chikungunya

Aftereffects	Households	Percentage
Yes	161	62.4
No	97	37.6
Total	258	100.0

More than three fifth (62.4 percent) of the households have members affected by Chikungunya witnessed after effects. These effects not only influenced their productivity thereby the income but also higher cost of illness due to prolonged illness. Table 7.17 shows the distribution of households according to the number of people affected on the basis of marital status.

Table 7.17: Number of members affected on the basis of marital status

Married members	Households	Percentage
One	138	57.3
Two	95	39.4
Three	7	2.9
Four	1	.4
Total	241	100.0
Unmarried members	**Households**	**Percentage**
One	28	84.8
Two	5	15.2
Total	33	100.0

It is found that 57.3 percent of the households having married members showing a single person affected as compared to 84.8 percent of the unmarried members in this category. In no household more than two unmarried members are affected by Chikungunya fever, whereas 2.9 and 0.4 percentages respectively of the households have two and three married members in this category.

Type of Medical Assistance

The type of medical service received by the sample household is shown in Table 7.18.

Table 7.18: Source of medical treatment

Source	Households	Percentage
private	203	78.7
public	46	17.8
both	9	3.5
Total	258	100.0

The survey revealed that 78.7 percent of the households depended on private medical practitioners for medical treatment. Only 17.2 percent of the sample households utilised public medical facilities for treating the disease. There are as many as 9 households (3.5 percent) utilised both private and public health care facilities for treating the disease.

It is observed that Kanyakumari District has medical centres for all types of treatment. People generally prefer Allopathy treatment for immediate cure. Ayurvedic and Sidha ways of treatment are for certain special health problems. Chikungunya fever patients visited Allopathy for recovery from fever and the aftermath effects are generally treated through Ayurvedic and Sidha methods.

Table 7.19 presents the descriptive statistics of the type of medical treatment. Allopathy is the type of medical treatment taken by 95.74 percent (247 out of 258) of the households having an average of 1.4 persons with a standard deviation of 0.697. Homeopathy, Ayurvedic and Sidha are the other types of treatments taken by 2.71, 1.94 and 1.63 percentages respectively of the total households. Majority of the households practiced Allopathy. Ayurveda and Sidha are adopted by the households to relieve from the after effects of Chikungunya. The latter types of treatment warrant longer period to cure hence side effects cost relatively high.

Table 7.19: Descriptive statistics of type of treatment

Type of treatment	Households	Minimum	Maximum	Mean	Std. Deviation
Allopathic	247	1.00	4.00	1.368	.6969
Homeopathy	7	1.00	3.00	2.142	1.0690
Sidha	3	1.00	2.00	1.333	.5773
Ayurvedic	5	1.00	1.00	1.000	.0000

The respondents were asked about the reasons why they selected a particular type of treatment. The answers given were classified in Table 7.20.

Table 7.20: Reason for selecting the treatment

Reasons	Households	Percentage
Cures better than any other treatment	149	57.8
Most neighbours select this source	81	31.4
Don't have money to choose any other source	22	8.5
others	6	2.3
Total	258	100.0

More respondents are quite reasonable in selecting the type of treatment. Out of 258 households, 57.8 percent selected the type of treatment because they know that it cures better than any other type of treatment. While a sizeable number of households selected a particular type of treatment because of the demonstration effect. They felt that the type of treatment they have taken because their 'neighbours have taken the same type of treatment'. This group constitutes 31.4 percent of the total households. The economic reason comprises a relatively lesser share of the households. The reason of 'do not have money to any other types of treatment' was the answer of 8.5 percent of the households.

The sick persons in some of the sample households suffer from some permanent or non-communicable health problems. Such patients have more probability of getting side effects. The descriptive statistics of sick persons of Chikungunya fever having some other non-communicable health problem is shown in Table 7.21.

Table 7.21: Descriptive statistics of other health problems

Other health problems	Households	Minimum	Maximum	Mean	Std. Deviation
Blood pressure	36	1.00	2.00	1.166	.3779
Diabetes	49	1.00	2.00	1.102	.3058
Ulcer	16	1.00	1.00	1.000	.0000
Arthritis	7	1.00	1.00	2.428	.7796
Tuberculosis	2	1.00	1.00	1.000	.0000

Diabetes is the most prominent non- communicable disease of the sick person affected by Chikungunya fever. Such households account for 18.99 percent (49 of 258) of the total households with an average of 1.1persons and standard deviation of 0.306. The problem of blood pressure was the case of 13.95 percent (36 out of 258) of the households having an average of 1.17 persons and standard deviation of 0.378. Ulcer, Arthritis and Tuberculosis are the other health problems of the households accounting for 6.59, 2.71 and 0.78 percentages respectively of the households. But all these households have a maximum of a single sick person in the respective health categories.

Problem of Sleeplessness

Sleeplessness is one of the important symptoms of Chikungunya fever. Sleeplessness was the problem of Chikungunya affected people during the period of illness. The distribution of households according to the number of patients with the problem of sleeplessness is shown in Table 7.22.

Table 7.22: Problem of sleeplessness during the fever

Number with sleeplessness problem	Households	Percentage
One	158	68.4
Two	54	23.4
Three	14	6.1
Four	5	2.2
Total	231	100.0

It is found that among the total households having patients expressed sleeplessness, 68.4 percent have a single person in this category. Households having two, three and four sick persons experienced sleeplessness problem are in the proportions of 23.4, 6.1 and 2.2 percentages respectively. It confirms that sleeplessness is an important symptom of Chikungunya fever among patients in the study area.

Chikungunya fever had been repeating in the study area continuously since 2006. Hence the respondents were asked about the repetition of the fever in their households. The results are furnished in Table 7.23. It is interesting to note that out of the 258 households only 10.9 percent experienced repetition of the fever in their households after 2006. There prevailed a general belief that once Chikungunya fever infected, the person has a rare possibility of infecting the fever again. None of the Chikungunya affected person experienced the repetition of the disease.

Table 7.23: Previous occurrence of Chikungunya fever

Previous occurrence	Households	Percentage
Yes	28	10.9
No	230	89.1
Total	258	100.0

Consulting Doctor

Consulting doctor for and illness is not a regular affair of poor people. They consult doctors only when the disease causes some kind of fear and uncertainty over the recovery. Hence the respondents were asked about consulting doctors. The details of doctor consultation are shown in Table 7.24.

Table 7.24: Consulted doctor

Consulted doctor	Households	Percentage
Yes	253	98.1
No	5	1.9
Total	258	100.0

It is quite interesting to note that 98.1 percent (253 of 258) households consulted doctors for curing Chikungunya fever affected members. It vividly clarifies that Chikungunya fever caused panic among the households in the study area. In some of the households, Chikungunya affected members developed some complications while treating the fever. Table 7.25 shows the presence of complicated cases among the sample households.

Table 7.25: Experience of complication

Complication	Households	Percentage
Yes	55	21.3
No	203	78.7
Total	258	100.0

It is reported that 21.3 percent of the households faced the difficulties of the Chikungunya fever developing complications. But four- fifth (78.7 percent) of the households opined that they did not face any complications in the treatment of the disease.

Time of Treatment

Time of taking the patient to doctors is one of the important measures to avoid complications arising out of a disease. The descriptive statistics of the time of treatment given to the patients by the households is presented in Table 7.26.

Table 7.26: Descriptive statistics of time of treatment

Time of treatment	Households	Minimum	Maximum	Mean	Std. Deviation
As soon as felt it	196	1.00	5.00	1.4337	.73078
When not allowed for work	46	1.00	4.00	1.3478	.67387
When it is serious	29	1.00	3.00	1.3103	.54139

It is found that 196 of the 258 (75.97 percent) households had taken their patients to doctors as soon as they felt the symptom of Chikungunya fever. However, 17.83 percent (46 households) of the households did the same when the fever not allowed them to do the regular job. Moreover, 11.24 percent (29 households) households consulted doctors only when the disease became very serious.

The reason for the late medical care is shown in Table 7.27.

Out of the 70 households given late medical care to the members affected by Chikungunya fever opined that 38.6 percent (27 households) could not take the patients to the doctors because they cannot afford such treatment immediately. It took some time for them to arrange finance for treatment. Over crowdedness in hospitals is cited as the second most important reason. It account for 24.3 percent (17 households). It is surprising to note that 17.1 percent of the households could not be given immediate treatment to the patients.

Table 7.27: Reason for late medical care

Reason	Households	Percentage
Clinics and hospital away from house	4	5.7
Over crowdedness in hospital	17	24.3
Cannot afford	27	38.6
No one to take to hospital	12	17.1
Others	10	14.3
Total	70	100.0

Immediate treatment could not be given to the patients because no one was available in their family to take them to the hospital. Distance or clinics and hospitals away from their house were the answer of 5.7 percent of the households given late medical care.

Sick Period

In order to understand the sick period of the Chikungunya affected people at the household level is classified into time to recover from fever, time taken for normalcy, suffering period of sickness and suffering period due to side effects or after effects. The descriptive statistics of the sick period of the sick members at the household level is furnished in Table 7.28.

It is evident that the average time taken to recover from the Chikungunya fever is 13.12 days for 258 households. The minimum is of 1day to a maximum of 200 days with a standard deviation of 18.344. The average time taken for normalcy is 50.97 days. The average suffering period of 139.05 days is lower than the average suffering period due to side effects of 190.25 days. This is the extent of acuteness of the fever in the study area. Many respondents still feel that their members did not become alright or cannot perform work to the same level prior to the infection of the fever even at the time of the survey.

Table 7.28: Descriptive statistics of sick period

Sick period (days/year)	Households	Minimum	Maximum	Mean	Std. Deviation
Time to recover from fever	258	1.00	200.00	13.124	18.3441
Time to bring normalcy	257	3.00	730.00	50.972	68.4065
Suffering period of illness	244	.00	1460.00	139.053	211.0535
Period of suffering due to side effects	256	.00	1460.00	190.257	268.0570

The survey revealed that many victims of Chikungunya fever shifted their occupation to less physically involving occupations. The opinion of households about their members taking the work load in the current period as compared to the same before the infection of Chikungunya fever is shown in Table 7.29.

Table 7.29: Doing the same work load as before

Ability of the sick person to carry previous workload	Households	Percentage
Yes	104	40.3
No	154	59.7
Total	258	100.0

Only two- fifth (40.3 percent) of the households responded that their members take the same work load as before. While the remaining three – fifth (59.7 percent) of the households have members affected by Chikungunya cannot be able to take the same work load as before because of the infection of the fever. Medical practitioners claim that fever is not a disease but only a symptom. Most of other fever patients recover from their illness within a short duration and take time taken to resilient their productivity. However, Chikungunya fever drastically reduced the labour productivity considerably for a long period.

Table 7.30 presents the particulars about change of occupation in sample households after the infection of Chikungunya fever.

Table 7.30: Change of occupation after Chick fever

Change of occupation	Households	Percentage
Yes	57	22.1
No	201	77.9
Total	258	100.0

It is interesting to see that though the efficiency of the people reduced after the Chikungunya fever in many households, only 22.1 percent of the households reported that they have members' changed their occupation after the fever.

Type of Patient

The sick persons of Chikungunya fever can be classified in to inpatient, outpatient and both. Inpatients are those consult doctors in a clinic or hospital and admit in hospital for treatment till they recover from fever. Outpatients go to a doctor, clinic or hospital to get consultation and prescription of medicines. Some households have members in both category or each member perform both as an inpatient and as an outpatient in the course of treatment. The details of different types of patients at the household level is shown in Table 7.31

Table 7.31: Type of patient

Type of patient	Households	Percentage
Inpatient	24	9.4
Outpatient	176	69.3
Both	54	21.3
Total	254	100.0

It is found that 69.3 percent of the sample households have outpatients. Both inpatients and outpatients form 21.3 percent. Only 9.4 percent of the households have inpatients. From Table 7.31 it is clear that 254 of the 258 households (98.45 percent) sought medical assistance to treat the sick people.

Mere medical assistance may not reveal the treating of the disease. Table 7.32 gives number of doctor's visit by each household and the distribution of the households according to the number of doctor's visits.

Table 7.32: Number of visits to doctor

No. of doctors visits	Households	Percentage
Less than 2	120	47.4
2 - 4	61	24.1
4 - 6	29	11.5
6 - 8	20	7.9
More than 8	23	9.1
Total	253	100.0

Out of 253 households consulted doctors, 47.4 percent made only a single visit. The pattern of distribution explains that lesser number of households is represented in the higher ranges of doctor consultations. Households made 2-4 visits account for 24.1 percent. It is noteworthy that 9.1 percent households made more than 8 doctor visits. Generally increased number of doctor visits is associated with the continuance of the illness or its side effects.

Cost of Illness

In order to assess the total cost of illness at the household level, both direct and indirect costs of illness are taken into account. Direct costs include those costs directly associated with the health care intervention. The present study has taken into account doctor's fee, costs of conducting medical tests, cost of medicines and transportation costs for the direct cost. Direct cost of inpatient includes all the items of cost to the outpatient plus accommodation cost. The indirect costs are the costs that are not directly accountable. Among the indirect costs, the wage losses to the sick person and caretaker are only taken into account. The wage loss also includes the loss suffered by the sick person due to the after effects of the disease. Intangible costs are not measured but described for the purpose of getting more insight into the intensity of the disease.

Direct Costs of Outpatient

The descriptive statistics of various components of the direct costs of the outpatients are shown in Table 7.33.

Table 7.33: Descriptive statistics of outpatient cost of illness

Outpatient- direct cost of illness	Households	Minimum	Maximum	Mean	Std. Deviation
Doctors fee (Rs)	177	30.00	15000.00	753.497	1604.891
Costs of tests(Rs)	130	25.00	3000.00	422.192	519.986
Costof medicines(Rs)	168	30.00	14000.00	1059.851	1716.166
Transportation cost(Rs)	187	10.00	1000.00	207.422	226.179

It is found that some patients are outpatients all along and some patients have acted both outpatient and inpatient. In the direct cost calculation of outpatients, the costs of latter class are taken in to account. Among the total households, 68.61 percent (177) households paid doctor fee as outpatient by paying a minimum of Rs.30 and to the maximum of Rs.15,000. The average doctor's fee of the households with outpatient is Rs.753.50 with a standard deviation of 1604.891. The average cost of medicines appears the highest of Rs.1059.85. But 65.12 percent of the households paid for medicines to their outpatients. The average cost of medicine and transportation of the households with outpatients are Rs.422.19 and Rs.207.42 respectively. Maximum number (187 out of 258 or 72.48 percent) of households incurred transportation cost and minimum number of households (130 out of 258 or 50.39 percent) have shown expenditure for tests.

Inpatient Direct Costs

Many of the sample households are outpatients because of the problem of getting admission to hospitals or medical centres as inpatients. Out of the total number of households having inpatients (74 out of 258 or 28.68 percent), 81.1 percent expressed that they faced problems in getting admissions into hospitals as inpatients. (Table 7.34).

Table 7.34: Problem in getting admission for indoor treatment

Problem	Households	Percentage
Yes	60	81.1
No	14	18.9
Total	74	100.0

The descriptive statistics of the cost of illness of the inpatient-households is shown in Table 7.35.

Among the different components of direct cost of illness, average accommodation and medicine costs of inpatient households are the largest. The average accommodation and medicine cost arrived at is Rs.1796.81.

Table 7.35: Descriptive statistics of inpatient cost of illness

Cost items	Households	Minimum	Maximum	Mean	Std. Deviation
Doctors fee (Rs)	74	50.00	8000.00	642.500	973.260
Diagnostic tests (Rs)	51	12.00	6000.00	674.156	969.298
Accommodation (Rs)	69	100.00	7500.00	1796.816	1669.293
Transportation (Rs)	70	30.00	4000.00	273.571	504.478

The second and third ranking components of cost of illness are diagnostic costs and doctor's fee accounting for Rs.674.16 and Rs.642.50 respectively. Transportation cost of inpatients is slightly higher than that of the same of outpatients because caretakers travel between residences and the hospitals many times till the patient is discharged from hospital.

Another important inference is that all the inpatients did not incur an expenditure on different components of cost of illness. Households paid doctors fees numbered more than transportation cost, accommodation and medicine and diagnostic tests. It is interesting to note that diagnostic tests are not available for Chikungunya in any of the hospitals in the study area but as many as 51 households having in patients(51 out of 78 or 65.38 percent) paid money for the purpose of conducting tests.

Indirect Cost

Wage loss of the patients and caretakers in the category of both outpatient and inpatient in a household is collectively termed as indirect cost. No other indirect cost is taken in the study because of the problem of the difficulty of accurate measurement. Table 7.36 furnishes the descriptive statistics of indirect cost of illness.

Wage loss to the sick persons is reported in 149 of the 258 (57.75 percent) households. Wage loss due to the side effects of Chikungunya fever is recorded in122 of the 258 (47.28 percent) households. Only 23 of the 258 (8.91 percent) witnessed wage loss to the care takers.

Table 7.36: Descriptive statistics of indirect cost of illness

Cost items	Households	Minimum	Maximum	Mean	Std. Deviation
Wage loss to the sick person	149	350.00	30000.00	3448.6577	4175.058
Wage loss to the caretaker	23	.00	8000.00	1691.3043	1777.041
Wage loss due to side effects	122	600.00	170000.00	5863.9344	15575.945

The average wage loss is the highest in the case of wage loss due to side effects. It is almost twice as that of the wage loss of the sick persons during the period of sickness. Anyhow wage loss to the care takers is not substantial when compared to the sick persons.

Total Cost of Illness

The distribution of households according to the level of total cost of illness is shown in Table 7.37.

It is found that one- third (32.6 percent) of the households incur an expenditure of less than Rs.2000. The next largest number of households is found in the expenditure class of Rs 4000- Rs 6000. They accounted for 14 percent of the households. The total cost of illness in the highest slab of above Rs.14000 comprises 12.8 percent of the households.

Table 7.37: Total cost of illness

Cost of illness	Households	Percentage
Less than 2000	84	32.6
2000 - 4000	34	13.2
4000 - 6000	36	14.0
6000 - 8000	31	12.0
8000 - 10000	24	9.3
10000 - 12000	6	2.3
12000 - 14000	10	3.9
Above 14000	33	12.8
Total	258	100.0

The experience of Chikungunya fever in sample households revealed that majority of them are affected with a single member. More than one-third of them managed the disease by incurring the lowest COI. The households affected the worst are the households where the wage earners affected. Lack of experience of the medical people caused complications in treatment. Side effects of the people in the working age group have eaten a large proportion of their income and their income generating ability.

Analysis Of Cost Of Illness Of Chikungunya Fever At The Household Level In Kanyakumari District

The rapid growth of mosquitoes in living environment increases the incidences of infectious diseases like the Chikungunya fever. Medical expenditure in treating Chikungunya fever, lost wages, defensive expenditure to prevent the diseases, the disutility arising out of the intensity of the disease and the lost opportunities of leisure are quantifiable. In the previous chapter the total cost of illness of Chikungunya fever at the household level is estimated. The present chapter analyses the total cost of illness of Chikungunya fever at the household level with various socio economic, demographic and other variables. An attempt is also made to analyse the determinants of the cost of illness, the probability of the penetration of the diseases among wage earners and the determinants of the incidence of the cost of illness of Chikungunya fever.

Socio Economic Determinants of Household Cost of Illness.

1. Age of the Head of the Household

This distribution of cost of illness according to the age of the head of the household is shown in Table 8.1.

It is evident that the total cost of illness of young and very old respondents headed households is found in the lower cost classes. More than two –thirds (66.7 percent) of the young respondents who are below 25 years of age and 80 percent of the very old aged above 75 years are found in the lowest total cost of illness class of less than Rs 2000. It is noteworthy that the households of respondents aged between 25 and 50 years of age are found more in the higher classes of the total cost of illness. For this age group, less than one fourth of the households (24.5 percent) are found in the lowest total cost of illness class. Households of respondents aged between 50 and 75 years of age have relatively more representation in the higher levels of total cost of illness.

Table 8.1: Distribution of total cost of illness according to the age of the respondent

Total cost of illness (in Rs)	Age of the respondent (in years)				Total
	Below 25	25-50	50-75	Above 75	
Less than 2000	4 (66.7)	36 (24.5)	40 (40.0)	4 (80.0)	84 (32.6)
2000 -4000	0 (0)	20 (13.6)	13 (13.0)	1 (20.0)	34 (13.2)
4000 -6000	1 (16.7)	18 (12.2)	17 (17.0)	0 (0)	36 (14.0)
6000 -8000	0 (0)	23 (15.6)	8 (8.0)	0 (0)	31 (12.0)
8000 -10000	0 (0)	16 (10.9)	8 (8.0)	0 (0)	24 (9.3)
10000 -12000	0 (0)	4 (2.7)	2 (2.0)	0 (0)	6 (2.3)
12000 -14000	0 (0)	7 (4.8)	3 (3.0)	0 (0)	10 (3.9)
Above 14000	1 (16.7)	23 (15.6)	9 (9.0)	0 (0)	33 (12.8)
Total	6 (100.0)	147 (100.0)	100(100.0)	5 (100.0)	258(100.0)

Note: Figures in the parentheses show column percentages

The young and very old respondents are relatively insignificant among the sample households. The respondents aged between 25 and 50 years have around 50 percent of the households in the total cost of illness class of Rs.6000 and above. They incur more expenditure for treating the Chikungunya fever because most of such households have sick persons in the working age group.

2. Sex

The distribution of cost of illness according to the sex of the respondents is furnished in Table 8.2.

Table 8.2: Distribution of total cost of illness
according to the sex of the respondent

Total cost of illness (in Rs.)	Sex		Total
	Male	Female	
Less than 2000	65 (31.6)	19 (36.5)	84 (32.6)
2000 -4000	25 (12.1)	9 (17.3)	34 (13.2)
4000 -6000	30 (14.6)	6 (11.5)	36 (14.0)
6000 -8000	24 (11.7)	7 (13.5)	31 (12.0)
8000 -10000	21 (10.2)	3 (5.8)	24 (9.3)
10000-12000	4 (1.9)	2 (3.8)	6 (2.3)
12000 -14000	10 (4.9)	0 (0)	10 (3.9)
Above 14000	27 (13.1)	6 (11.5)	33 (12.8)
Total	206 (100.0)	52(100.0)	258 (100.0)

Note: Figures in the parentheses show column percentages

The female headed households show no substantial difference in the total cost of illness when compared to the male headed households. In the lowest two classes of the total cost of illness, the percentage share of women headed households are more. In the higher classes of cost of illness except in Rs.6000-8000 and Rs.10000-12000, the percentage share of households belonging to the male headed households have more representation. It can be inferred that the percentage share of female headed households are more in the lower classes of total cost of illness.

3. Communities

Table 8.3 presents the distribution of total cost of illness according to the communities.

Table 8.3: Distribution of total cost of illness according to community

Total cost of illness(in Rs)	Community					
	Scheduled Caste	Scheduled Tribe	Most Backward Class	Backward Class	Others	Total
Less than 2000	8 (40.0)	0 (0)	5 (62.5)	58 (29.1)	12 (42.9)	83 (32.3)
2000 - 4000	3 (15.0)	1 (50.0)	2 (25.0)	24 (12.1)	4 (14.3)	34 (13.2)
4000 - 6000	2 (10.0)	1 (50.0)	1 (12.5)	25 (12.6)	7 (25.0)	36 (14.0)
6000 - 8000	2 (10.0)	0 (0)	0 (0)	27 (13.6)	2 (7.1)	31 (12.1)
8000 - 10000	3 (15.0)	0 (0)	0 (0)	21 (10.6)	0 (0)	24 (9.3)
10000 -12000	1 (5.0)	0 (0)	0 (0)	4 (2.0)	1 (3.6)	6 (2.3)
12000 -14000	0 (0)	0 (0)	0 (0)	10 (5.0)	0 (0)	10 (3.9)
Above 14000	1 (5.0)	0 (0)	0 (0)	30 (15.1)	2 (7.1)	33 (12.8)
Total	20 (100.0)	2 (100.0)	8 (100.0)	199 (100.0)	28 (100.0)	257 (100.0)

Note: Figures in the parentheses show column percentages

It is interesting to note that the percentage share of Backward Class households is the least (29.1 percent) in the lowest class of total cost of illness though there is no representation of Scheduled Tribe households in this group. The share of Most Backward Class households in the lowest total cost of illness class is the highest consisting of 62.5 percent when compared to 40 percent of the Scheduled Caste households and 42.9 percent of the households in the category of others. The Backward Class households comprise mainly Christian and Hindu Nadars who have the highest representation in the highest class of total cost of illness. It is found that no household among the Scheduled Tribe and Most Backward Class is in the total cost of illness group above Rs.4000-6000. Backward Caste households represent relatively more in the upper classes of the total cost of illness.

4. Religion

Table 8.4 shows the distribution of cost of illness according to the religious composition of the households.

Table 8.4: Distribution of total cost of illness according to religious groups

Total cost of illness (in Rs.)	Religion				Total
	Hindu	Christian	Muslim	Others	
Less than 2000	30 (30.0)	52 (33.3)	1 (100.0)	1 (100.0)	84 (32.6)
2000 -4000	15 (15.0)	19 (12.2)	0 (0)	0 (0)	34 (13.2)
4000 -6000	14 (14.0)	22 (14.1)	0 (0)	0 (0)	36 (14.0)
6000 -8000	9 (9.0)	22 (14.1)	0 (0)	0 (0)	31 (12.0)
8000 -10000	9 (9.0)	15 (9.6)	0 (0)	0 (0)	24 (9.3)
10000 -12000	3 (3.0)	3 (1.9)	0 (0)	0 (0)	6 (2.3)
12000 -14000	5 (5.0)	5 (3.2)	0 (0)	0 (0)	10 (3.9)
Above 14000	15 (15.0)	18 (11.5)	0 (0)	0 (0)	33 (12.8)
Total	100 (100.0)	156 (100.0)	1 (100.0)	1 (100.0)	258 (100.0)

Note: Figures in the parentheses show column percentages

It is evident that Christian and Hindu households are predominant among the Chikungunya affected households. A Muslim household and a household in the category of others in the religious group are found in the lowest total cost of illness class. One third (33.3 percent) of the Christian households and 30 percent of the Hindu households represent in the lowest total cost of illness class. Nevertheless Hindu and Christian households in the highest total cost of illness class of above Rs.14 000 accounts for 15 and 11.5 percentages respectively. Though religion is not a direct factor influencing the cost of illness but the survey data show that Hindu households represent more in the higher total cost of illness classes.

5. Literacy Status

Studies on cost of illness explain that literacy is an important factor influencing the cost. The distribution of cost of illness according to the literacy status of the head of the household is given in Table 8.5.

Table 8.5: Distribution of total cost of illness according to literacy status

Total cost of illness (in Rs)	Literacy status		Total
	Literate	Illiterate	
Less than 2000	68 (30.5)	16 (45.7)	84 (32.6)
2000 -4000	27 (12.1)	7 (20.0)	34 (13.2)
4000 -6000	33 (14.8)	3 (8.6)	36 (14.0)
6000 -8000	29 (13.0)	2 (5.7)	31 (12.0)
8000 -10000	21 (9.4)	3 (8.6)	24 (9.3)
10000 -12000	5 (2.2)	1 (2.9)	6 (2.3)
12000 -14000	10 (4.5)	0 (0)	10 (3.9)
Above 14000	30 (13.5)	3 (8.6)	33 (12.8)
Total	223 (100.0)	35 (100.0)	258 (100.0)

Note: Figures in the parentheses show column percentages

The households of illiterate respondents have higher percentage share in the lowest classes of total cost of illness. Out of the 33 households of illiterate respondents, 65.7 percent of them are present in the classes of less than Rs.4000 category of the total cost of illness. But for literate households, the percentage share in the lowest two classes of total cost of illness is only 42.6. It is found that 18.0 percent of the households of the literate respondents represent in the highest total cost of illness classes of Rs. 12000-14000 and above Rs.14000 as compared to 8.6 percent of the same of the households of illiterate respondents. The general trend is that the literate respondents spend relatively more for defending the sickness.

6. Educational Standard

The distribution of the total cost of illness of the households according to the educational standard of the literate respondent is shown in Table 8.6.

A comparison of total cost of illness of the household according to the educational standard of the respondents revealed that 60 percent of the households of graduate respondents and 100 percent of the professionals are placed in the lowest total cost of illness class of less than Rs. 2000. Followed by professionals and graduate respondents, households of higher secondary school level educated respondents are found in the lowest total cost of illness accounting for 41.7 percent. The households of high school level educated respondents are found having the least share in the lowest class of total cost of illness. In the highest class of total cost of illness of above Rs.14000, the households of higher secondary level educated respondents share 29.2 percent. The households of school level educated respondents are found in almost all classes of total cost of illness whereas household of highly educated respondents are found more in the lower classes of total cost of illness.

7. Type of Family

The distribution of the total cost of illness according to the type of family is shown in Table 8.7.

Table 8.6: Distribution of educational standard of the respondents according to the total cost of illness

Educational standard	Total cost of illness (in Rs)								Total
	Less than 2000	2000 -4000	4000 -6000	6000 -8000	8000 -10000	10000 -12000	12000 -14000	Above 14000	
Primary school	17 (30.4)	8 (14.3)	6 (10.7)	7 (12.5)	4 (7.1)	1 (1.8)	5 (8.9)	8 (14.3)	56 (100.0)
Middle school	11 (31.4)	1 (2.9)	6 (17.1)	6 (17.1)	4 (11.4)	2 (5.7)	1 (2.9)	4 (11.4)	35 (100.0)
High school	17 (20.7)	14 (17.1)	18 (22.0)	11 (13.4)	10 (12.2)	2 (2.4)	2 (2.4)	8 (9.8)	82 (100.0)
Higher secondary	10 (41.7)	2 (8.3)	1 (4.2)	2 (8.3)	2 (8.3)	0 (0)	0 (0)	7 (29.2)	24 (100.0)
Graduates	9 (60.0)	0 (.0)	2 (13.3)	2 (8.3)	0 (.0)	0 (0)	0 (0)	2 (13.3)	15 (100.0)
Post graduates	2 (25.0)	2 (25.0)	0 (0)	0 (0)	1 (12.5)	0 (0)	2 (25.0)	1 (12.5)	8 (100.0)
Professional	2 (100.0)	0 (0)	0 (0)	0 (0)	0 (0)	0 (0)	0 (0)	0 (0)	2 (100.0)
Others	0 (0)	0 (0)	0 (0)	1 (100.0)	0 (0)	0 (0)	0 (0)	0 (0)	1 (100.0)
Total	68 (30.5)	27 (12.1)	33 (14.8)	29 (13.0)	21 (9.4)	5 (2.2)	10 (4.5)	30 (13.5)	223 (100.0)

Note: Figures in the parentheses show row percentages

Table 8.7: Distribution of total cost of illness
according to the type of family

Total cost of illness (in Rs)	Type of family			Total
	Nuclear	Joint	Uni-member	
Less than 2000	71 (31.8)	11 (35.5)	2 (50.0)	84 (32.6)
2000 -4000	25 (11.2)	7 (22.6)	2 (50.0)	34 (13.2)
4000 -6000	33 (14.8)	3 (9.7)	0 (0)	36 (14.0)
6000 -8000	28 (12.6)	3 (9.7)	0 (0)	31 (12.0)
8000 -10000	22 (9.9)	2 (6.5)	0 (0)	24 (9.3)
10000 -12000	6 (2.7)	0 (0)	0 (0)	6 (2.3)
12000 -14000	7 (3.1)	3 (9.7)	0 (0)	10 (3.9)
Above 14000	31 (13.9)	2 (6.5)	0 (0)	33 (12.8)
Total	223 (100.0)	31 (100.0)	4 (100.0)	258 (100.0)

Note: Figures in the parentheses show column percentages

It is interesting to note that 58.1 percent of the Joint families represent in the lowest total cost of illness class of less than Rs. 4000 as compared to 43 percent of the same of the nuclear families. All the uni-member households belong to the lowest two classes of total cost of illness. The percentage shares of nuclear families are more in the higher classes of total cost of illness. This is due to the fact that Chikungunya fever caused more problems in those households. The ratio of number of income earners to the total household size is less in the case of nuclear families hence the infection of Chikungunya fever caused more direct and indirect cost of illness to the nuclear type of households than any other type of families.

8. Occupation of the Respondent

Table 8.8 shows the distribution of total cost of illness of the households according to the occupation of the respondents.

Table 8.8: Total cost of illness according to the occupation of the respondent

Occupation	Total cost of illness								Total
	Less than 2000	2000 -4000	4000 -6000	6000 -8000	8000 -10000	10000 -2000	12000 -14000	Above 14000	
Labourers	28 (21.9)	19 (14.8)	26 (20.3)	19 (14.8)	14 (10.9)	3 (2.3)	4 (3.1)	15 (11.7)	128 (100.0)
Teacher	1 (14.3)	1 (14.3)	2 (28.6)	1 (14.3)	2 (28.6)	0 (0)	0 (0)	0 (0)	7 (100.0)
Soldier	5 (62.5)	1 (12.5)	0 (0)	1 (12.5)	1 (12.5)	0 (0)	0 (0)	0 (0)	8 (100.0)
Driver	3 (42.9)	2 (28.6)	0 (0)	1 (14.3)	0 (0)	0 (0)	0 (0)	1 (14.3)	7 (100.0)
Government Employee	7 (63.6)	1 (9.1)	2 (18.2)	0 (0)	0 (0)	0 (0)	1 (9.1)	0 (0)	11 (100.0)
Factory Worker	2 (40.0)	1 (20.0)	0 (0)	0 (0)	0 (0)	0 (0)	0 (0)	2 (40.0)	5 (100.0)
Agriculture	6 (40.0)	0 (0)	1 (6.7)	2 (13.3)	2 (13.3)	0 (0)	2 (13.3)	2 (13.3)	15 (100.0)
Tailor	0 (0)	0 (0)	0 (0)	0 (0)	0 (0)	0 (0)	0 (0)	1 (100.0)	1 (100.0)
Industrial Worker	6 (85.7)	0 (0)	0 (0)	0 (0)	0 (0)	0 (0)	0 (0)	1 (0)	7 (100.0)
Construction	3 (42.9)	0 (0)	1 (14.3)	1 (14.3)	1 (14.3)	0 (0)	0 (0)	1 (14.3)	7 (100.0)
Mason	2 (28.6)	1 (14.3)	0 (0)	1 (0)	0 (0)	1 (14.3)	1 (14.3)	1 (14.3)	7 (100.0)
Business	2 (22.2)	1 (11.1)	0 (0)	3 (33.3)	1 (11.1)	0 (0)	1 (11.1)	1 (11.1)	9 (100.0)
House Making	9 (42.9)	4 (19.0)	1 (4.8)	2 (9.5)	0 (0)	1 (4.8)	0 (0)	4 (19.0)	21 (100.0)
Fishing	6 (50.0)	1 (8.3)	2 (16.7)	0 (0)	1 (8.3)	1 (8.3)	1 (8.3)	0 (0)	12 (100.0)
Others	4 (30.8)	2 (15.4)	1 (7.7)	0 (0)	2 (15.4)	0 (0)	0 (0)	4 (30.8)	1 (100.0)
Total	84 (32.6)	34 (13.2)	36 (14.0)	31 (12.0)	24 (9.3)	6 (2.3)	10 (3.9)	33 (12.8)	258 (100.0)

Note: Figures in the parentheses show row percentages

It is evident that most of the households of formal employees are concentrated more in the lowest classes of the total cost of illness because absence of work during the sick period has less impact on their income generation. Households of most of the informal workers are the worst affected because in such households absence of work badly affect the process of their income generation. Informal workers mostly involved in occupations exerting more physical energy. It is observed during the survey that the household of a tailor was the worst affected. The head of the household was the victim of Chikungunya fever and the after effects of the diseases prolonged for a long period. He was the lone income earner of the family and the Chikungunya fever did not allow him perform his work for long. His family was indebted and the impact of the fever is severe for the family for quite a long period.

9. Size of Household

Large households have the possibility of more members affected due to the Chikungunya fever. The distribution of total cost of illness according to the size of household is shown in Table 8.9.

The comparison of the total cost of illness with regard to the size of the family presents that 41.7 percent households with two members are found in the lowest total cost of illness class of less than Rs. 2000 and the lowest share in this cost of illness class is the household size of seven members who account for 12.5 percent. The highest total cost of illness class of above Rs. 14000 comprises households having the family size between two and five. It is found that 17.1 percent of the households with four members record the maximum in the highest cost of illness class and 8.2 percent of the households with five members in this cost group. Another interesting feature is that households with a family size of three, four and five present more in the highest class of total cost of illness.

Table 8.9: Distribution of total cost of illness according to the household size

Total cost of illness (in Rs)	Household size								Total
	One	Two	Three	Four	Five	Six	Seven	Eight	
Less than 2000	1 (33.3)	15 (41.7)	15 (30.6)	33 (31.4)	16 (32.7)	1 (20.0)	1 (12.5)	2 (66.7)	84 (32.6)
2000 - 4000	2 (66.7)	1 (2.8)	6 (12.2)	14 (13.3)	5 (10.2)	3 (60.0)	3 (37.5)	0 (0)	34 (13.2)
4000 - 6000	0 (0)	8 (22.2)	5 (10.2)	9 (8.6)	11 (22.4)	1 (20.0)	2 (25.0)	0 (0)	36 (14.0)
6000 - 8000	0 (0)	1 (2.8)	8 (16.3)	17 (16.2)	5 (10.2)	0 (0)	0 (0)	0 (0)	31 (12.0)
8000 - 10000	0 (0)	4 (11.1)	6 (12.2)	7 (6.7)	5 (10.2)	0 (0)	1 (12.5)	1 (33.3)	24 (9.3)
10000 - 12000	0 (0)	1 (2.8)	2 (4.1)	2 (1.9)	1 (2.0)	0 (0)	0 (0)	0 (0)	6 (2.3)
12000 - 14000	0 (0)	0 (0)	2 (4.1)	5 (4.8)	2 (4.1)	0 (0)	1 (12.5)	0 (0)	10 (3.9)
Above 14000	0 (0)	6 (16.7)	5 (10.2)	18 (17.1)	4 (8.2)	0 (0)	0 (0)	0 (0)	33 (12.8)
Total	3 (100)	36 (100)	49 (100)	105 (100)	49 (100)	5 (100)	8 (100)	3 (100)	258 (100)

Note: Figures in the parentheses show column percentages

However, in the higher household size of six, seven and eight consist 100, 70.0 and 66.7 percentages respectively in the lower three classes of cost of illness. From this it can be inferred that households having lesser family size are intended to spend more to defend the sickness when compared to households having higher family size.

10. Monthly Household Income

Household income is one of the important determinants of the level of total cost of illness. High income households are ready to spend more on treating a disease. But poor people often find it difficult to get the minimum necessary treatment cost for even the chronic diseases. The distribution of the total cost of illness according their monthly household income is shown in Table 8.10.

It is found that 55.5 percent of the lowest income households are found in the lowest classes of total cost of sickness. However 33.3 percent of the lowest income households have incurred total cost of illness of Rs.8000-10000 and Rs.10000- 12000 comprising for 22.2 and 11.1 percentages respectively. In all the income classes except in the income class of Rs.10000-Rs.12500, maximum percentage of households are found in the lowest total cost of illness class of less than Rs.2000. However, in the highest total cost of illness class of above Rs.14000, 27.7 percent of the households having a monthly income of Rs.7501-10000 are present. All other income groups have percentage shares ranging from a minimum of zero percent to the maximum of 17.1 percent in this cost of illness class. In the highest total cost of illness class, higher income groups have more percentage share. However, higher income households are concentrated more in the lowest two classes of total cost of sickness.

Table 8.10: Distribution of total cost of illness according to the monthly household income

Total cost of illness (in Rs)	Total monthly household income (in Rs)								Total
	Below 2500	2501-5000	5001-7500	7501-10000	10001-12500	12501-15000	15501-17500	Above 17500	
Less than 2000	4 (44.4)	21 (38.9)	20 (33.9)	13 (27.7)	3 (23.1)	7 (30.4)	4 (33.3)	12 (29.3)	84 (32.6)
2000 - 4000	1 (11.1)	1 (1.9)	9 (15.3)	7 (14.9)	1 (7.7)	7 (30.4)	4 (33.3)	4 (9.8)	34 (13.2)
4000 - 6000	1 (11.1)	11 (20.4)	9 (15.3)	2 (4.3)	3 (23.1)	3 (13.0)	1 (8.3)	6 (14.6)	36 (14.0)
6000 - 8000	0 (0)	7 (13.0)	7 11.9	7 (14.9)	4 (30.8)	0 (0)	0 (0)	6 (14.6)	31 (12.0)
8000 - 10000	2 (22.2)	5 (9.3)	7 (11.9)	3 (6.4)	0 (0)	4 (17.4)	1 (8.3)	2 (4.9)	24 (9.3)
10000 - 12000	1 (11.1)	2 (3.7)	1 (1.7)	1 (2.1)	0 (0)	0 (0)	0 (0)	1 2.4	6 (2.3)
12000 - 14000	0 (0)	3 (5.6)	1 (1.7)	1 (2.1)	0 (0)	2 (8.7)	0 (0)	3 (7.3)	10 (3.9)
Above 14000	0 (0)	4 (7.4)	5 (8.5)	13 (27.7)	2 (15.4)	0 (0)	2 (16.7)	7 (17.1)	33 (12.8)
Total	9 (100)	54 (100)	59 (100)	47 (100)	13 (100)	23 (100)	12 (100)	41 (100)	258 (100)

Note: Figures in the parentheses show column percentages

Households in the higher income groups of Rs.12501 -15000 and Rs.15501 - 17500 consists of 66.6 and 60.8 percent respectively of the income groups in the lowest two classes of total cost of illness. It is observed that since most of the high income households are literates, they have better knowledge about treating the disease economically. They consulted government doctors and took rest and consumed liquid food without spending much on testing and medicines. Hence they are found more in the lower classes of total cost of illness. On the other hand, poor households are mostly engaged in informal employment. They were panic about the fever feeling similar to Malaria or Dengue and due to the fear psychosis of mortality they treated the disease at high cost even borrowing money at high interest rates.

11. Debt

Table 8.11 describes total cost of illness according to the level of household debt.

Out of the 184 indebted, 58 households (31.5 percent) are in the lowest total cost of illness class. In the highest total cost of illness class, the indebted households account for 15.2 percent. The total cost of illness across different levels of household debt reveal that in the category of the highest level of debtor households of above Rs.2 lakh, 43.8 percent belong to the least total cost of illness class of less than Rs.2000. However, debtor households in the category of Rs.25000-50000, Rs.100001-150000 and Rs.75001-100000 are in the percentages of 26.4, 28.6 and 20.0 respectively present in the highest total cost of illness class of above Rs.14 000. It is also found that more than one – fourth of the debtor households (28.8 percent) have a debt between 25,000- 50,000 of whom 26.4 percent are reported in the highest total cost of illness class of above Rs.14000.

Table 8.11: Total cost of illness according to household debt

Total cost of illness (in Rs.)	Household Debt								Total
	Below 25000	25001 -50000	50001 -75000	75001 -1000000	100001 -125000	125001 -150000	175001 -200000	Above 200000	
Less than 2000	14 (28.6)	20 (37.7)	4 (28.6)	7 (28.0)	3 (42.9)	2 (25.0)	1 (8.3)	7 (43.8)	58 (31.5)
2000 - 4000	6 (12.2)	3 (5.7)	2 (14.3)	2 (8.0)	0 (0)	0 (0)	4 (33.3)	2 (12.5)	19 (10.3)
4000 - 6000	12 (24.5)	4 (7.5)	2 (14.3)	3 (12.0)	0 (0)	0 (0)	1 (8.3)	1 (6.3)	23 (12.5)
6000 - 8000	6 (12.2)	4 (7.5)	3 (21.4)	1 (4.0)	2 (28.6)	2 (25.0)	2 (16.7)	3 (18.8)	23 (12.5)
8000 - 10000	5 (10.2)	4 (7.5)	2 (14.3)	4 (16.0)	0 (0)	3 (37.5)	1 (8.3)	0 (0)	19 (10.3)
10000 - 12000	1 (2.0)	2 (3.8)	0 (0)	1 (4.0)	0 (0)	0 (0)	0 (0)	1 (6.3)	5 (2.7)
12000 - 14000	3 (6.1)	2 (3.8)	0 (0)	2 (8.0)	0 (0)	1 (12.5)	1 (8.3)	0 (0)	9 (4.9)
Above 14000	2 (4.1)	14 (26.4)	1 (7.1)	5 (20.0)	2 (28.6)	0 (0)	2 (16.7)	2 (12.5)	28 (15.2)
Total	49 (100)	53 (100)	14 (100)	25 (100)	7 (100)	8 (100)	12 (100)	16 (100)	184 (100)

Note: Figures in the parentheses show column percentages

It is found that the households in the higher debt classes borrowed money more for various non-medical purposes. On the other, households in the lower classes of indebtedness mostly indulged in debts to treat their disease and to face the economic contingencies as a result of wage loss.

12. Area of the House

Table 8.12 shows the distribution of the total cost of illness of households according to the area of the house.

Table 8.12: Total cost of illness according to total area of the house

Total cost of illness (in Rs)	Total area of the house (in sq.ft)				Total
	Below 500	501 -750	751 -1000	Above 1000	
Less than 2000	12 (19.7)	31 (35.6)	27 (32.9)	14 (50.0)	84 (32.6)
2000 - 4000	9 (14.8)	10 (11.5)	12 (14.6)	3 (10.7)	34 (13.2)
4000 - 6000	10 (16.4)	14 (16.1)	10 (12.2)	2 (7.1)	36 (14.0)
6000 - 8000	8 (13.1)	10 (11.5)	8 (9.8)	5 (17.9)	31 (12.0)
8000 - 10000	8 (13.1)	9 (10.3)	6 (7.3)	1 (3.6)	24 (9.3)
10000 - 12000	2 (3.3)	2 (2.3)	1 (1.2)	1 (3.6)	6 (2.3)
12000 - 14000	5 (8.2)	2 (2.3)	3 (3.7)	0 (0)	10 (3.9)
Above 14000	7 (11.5)	9 (10.3)	15 (18.3)	2 (7.1)	33 (12.8)
Total	61 (100)	87 (100)	82(100)	28 (100)	258 (100)

Note: Figures in the parentheses show column percentages

It is evident that half (50 percent) of the households living in houses having the largest area above 1000 sq.ft present in the lowest level of cost of illness of less than Rs.2000 as compared to a mere 19.7 percent of the households in the same total cost of illness class living in houses having the lowest housing area of below 500 sq.ft. Most of the households living in the larger houses are found in the lower classes of the total cost of illness whereas more households living in the smaller houses are found relatively less in the lower total cost of illness classes. Households in larger houses of 751-1000 sq.ft and above 1000 sq.ft share 76.5 and 85.7 percent of their respective total households in the lower four classes of total cost of illness as compared to 74.7 and 64 percentages of the households in smaller houses of 501 to 750 sq.ft and 500 sq.ft and below respectively. Though area of the houses has no direct relationship with the cost of illness, it can be taken as an indicator of the severity of infection of Chikungunya in households. It is observed that households living in larger houses have better coping strategies to prevent the entry of mosquitoes. Hence the infection rate is very low among them.

13. Access Way to the House

Table 8.13 shows the distribution of total cost of illness according to the access way to the houses of the respondents.

The access way to the houses can be arranged according to the order of convenience in the descending order as vehicular road, paved path, unpaved path and others. It can be seen that no household in the category of others is seen in the lower four classes of the total cost of illness. However, the percentage share of households who has access way to their houses in the category of vehicular road, paved path and unpaved path in the lower four classes of total cost of illness are 68.8, 74.5 and 76.5 respectively. From this it is clear that households have better quality of access way to the houses are found less in the lower classes of total cost of illness.

Table 8.13: Total cost of illness according to access way to the house

Total cost of illness (in Rs)	Access way to the house				Total
	Vehicular road	Paved path	Unpaved path	Others	
Less than 2000	38 (31.1)	40 (36.4)	6 (25.0)	0 (0)	84 (32.6)
2000 - 4000	18 (14.8)	12 (10.9)	4 (16.7)	0 (0)	34 (13.2)
4000 - 6000	16 (13.1)	16 (14.5)	4 (16.7)	0 (0)	36 (14.0)
6000 - 8000	12 (9.8)	14 (12.7)	5 (20.8)	0 (0)	31 (12.0)
8000 - 10000	12 (9.8)	9 (8.2)	2 (8.3)	1 (50.0)	24 (9.3)
10000 - 12000	4 (3.3)	1 (.9)	1 (4.2)	0 (0)	6 (2.3)
12000 - 14000	7 (5.7)	2 (1.8)	1 (4.2)	0 (0)	10 (3.9)
Above 14000	15 (12.3)	16 (14.5)	1 (4.2)	1 (50.0)	33 (12.8)
Total	122 (100)	110 (100)	24 (100)	2 (100)	258 (100)

Note: Figures in the parentheses show column percentages

14. Distance between Residence and Vehicular Path

The distribution of cost of illness according to the distance between their residence and vehicular road is shown in Table 8.14.

The survey data have shown that 57.8 percent of the households (149 out of 258) reside at a distance less than 200 metres from the vehicular road. Out of the 149 households reside less than 200 metres from the vehicular road, 34.9 percent have the total cost of illness less than Rs.2000. The next highest share of 14.8 percent of the households residing in houses having a distance of less than 200 metres from the vehicular road represent in the highest total cost of illness class of above Rs.14000. More than one-fourth (27.8 percent) of the households in the category of having 200 – 400 metres represented the maximum in the total cost of illness class of above Rs.14000 Relatively more households having larger distance from the vehicular road is found in the higher classes of the total cost of illness.

Table 8.14: Total cost of illness according to distance between residence and vehicular path

Total cost of illness (in Rs)	Distance between residence and vehicular path (in metres)							Total
	Below 200	200 -400	400 -600	600 -800	800 -1000	Above 1000		
Less than 2000	52 (34.9)	7 (38.9)	5 (19.2)	4 (40.0)	9 (28.1)	7 (30.4)		84 (32.6)
2000 - 4000	18 (12.1)	0 (0)	7 (26.9)	3 (30.0)	2 (6.3)	4 (17.4)		34 (13.2)
4000 - 6000	16 (10.7)	1 (5.6)	8 (30.8)	1 (10.0)	7 (21.9)	3 (13.0)		36 (14.0)
6000 - 8000	19 12.8)	3 (16.7)	1 (3.8)	0 (0)	4 (12.5)	4 (17.4)		31 (12.0)
8000 - 10000	13 (8.7)	2 (11.1)	3 (11.5)	1 (10.0)	4 (12.5)	1 (4.3)		24 (9.3)
10000 - 12000	3 (2.0)	0 (0)	1 (3.8)	0 (0)	1 (3.1)	1 (4.3)		6 (2.3)
12000 - 14000	6 (4.0)	0 (0)	0 (0)	0 (0)	3 (9.4)	1 (4.3)		10 (3.9)
Above 14000	22 (14.8)	5 (27.8)	1 (3.8)	1 (10.0)	2 (6.3)	2 (8.7)		33 (12.8)
Total	149 (100)	18 (100)	26 (100)	10 (100)	32 (100)	23 (100)		258 (100)

Note: Figures in the parentheses show column percentages

15. Members Affected by Chikungunya in Households

The distribution of total cost of illness according to households with number of members affected is shown in Table 8.15

Table 8.15: Total cost of illness according to the number of members affected by Chikungunya in households

Total cost of illness (in Rs)	Number of members affected by Chikungunya					Total
	One	Two	Three	Four	Five	
Less than 2000	68 (43.0)	9 (13.8)	7 (26.9)	0 (0)	0 (0)	84 (32.6)
2000 - 4000	22 (13.9)	5 (7.7)	5 (19.2)	2 (25.0)	0 (0)	34 (13.2)
4000 - 6000	18 (11.4)	14 (21.5)	4 (15.4)	0 (0)	0 (0)	36 (14.0)
6000 - 8000	11 (7.0)	14 (21.5)	4 (15.4)	2 (25.0)	0 (0)	31 (12.0)
8000 - 10000	13 (8.2)	7 (10.8)	3 (11.59)	1 (12.5)	0 (0)	24 (9.3)
10000 - 12000	3 (1.9)	3 (4.6)	0 (0)	0 (0)	0 (0)	6 (2.3)
12000 - 14000	3 (12.7)	5 (7.7)	0 (11.5)	2 (25.0)	0 (0)	10 (3.9))
Above - 14000	20 (12.66)	8 (12.3)	3 (11.5)	1 (12.5)	1 (100)	33 (12.8)
Total	158 (100)	65 (100)	26 (100)	6(100)	1(100)	258 (100)

Note: Figures in the parentheses show column percentages

More than two-fifth (43 percent) of the households with single member affected have the least total cost of illness of less than Rs.2000. Among the households with two members affected by Chikungunya fever, 43 percent of them are present in the total cost of illness classes of Rs. 4000 – Rs 6000 and Rs. 6000 – 8000 having a share of 21.5 percent each. It is interesting to note that households with three members affected comprise 26.9 percent in the lowest total cost of illness class of less than Rs.2000 and 76.9 of them in the first four classes of the total cost of illness. There exists a lesser degree of direct correlation between cost of illness and number of household members affected by Chikungunya. It is noteworthy that most of the households present in the highest class of total cost of illness belong to the households with less number of people affected by Chikungunya fever.

16. Wage Earners Affected

The distribution of cost of illness according to the wage earners affected households by Chikungunya fever is shown in Table 8.16.

Table 8.16: Total cost of illness according to wage earners affected

Total cost of illness (in Rs.)	Wage earners affected households		Total
	Yes	No	
Less than 2000	36 (21.6)	48 (52.7)	84 (32.6)
2000 - 4000	18 (10.8)	16 (17.6)	34 (13.2)
4000 - 6000	23 (13.8)	13 (14.3)	36 (14.0)
6000 - 8000	27 (16.2)	4 (4.4)	31 (12.0)
8000 - 10000	21 (12.6)	3 (3.3)	24 (9.3)
10000 - 12000	6 (3.6)	0 (0)	6 (2.3)
12000 - 14000	9 (5.4)	1 (1.1)	10 (3.9)
Above 14000	27 (16.2)	6 (6.6)	33 (12.8)
Total	167 (100)	91 (100)	258 (100)

Note: Figures in the parentheses show column percentages

It is quite evident that more than half (52.7 percent) of the households having no wage earners affected are placed in the lowest total cost of illness class of less than Rs.2000. Only 11 percent of the no wage earner affected households are found in the higher total cost of illness classes of Rs.8000 and more. Whereas 37.8 percent of the wage earner affected households are present in the higher total cost of illness classes of Rs.8000 and more. Only one-fifth of the (21.6 percent) wage earner affected households represented in the lowest total cost of illness class. The pattern of the distribution of total household cost of illness among the sample households reveal that number of wage earner affected households are found less when go up in the total cost of illness classes, while more percentage share of wage- earner affected households are found in higher classes of total cost of illness.

17. Medical Expenses

Management of medical expense during the period of health crisis is severe in the case of households in the poor socio- economic order. Hence the management of finance necessary to treat the Chikungunya fever with the total cost of illness of the sample households was examined. The reported answers are furnished in Table.8.17.

The distribution of total cost of illness according to the management of medical expenses revealed that out of the 48.5 percent (125 out of 258) of the households borrowed money from various sources to treat the disease, more than one – fourth (25.6 percent) belongs to the lowest class of total illness cost of less than Rs.2000. The next largest two groups of households are found in the total cost of illness classes of Rs.6000 – 8000 and above Rs.14000 accounting for the percentages of 16.8 and 13.6 respectively. The second largest group of 97 households out of 258 (37.6 percent) managed finance for treating the disease from their own savings. Nearly two–fifth (39.2 percent) of such households represent the lowest total cost of illness class of below Rs.2000 and four out of every five (81.5 percent) household is found in the lower cost of illness classes below Rs. 8000. Hence it is clear that households depend on savings for treating the disease incurred less total cost of illness. It is found that two – third (66.6 percent) of the households depend on friends and relatives for meeting the expenditure for treatment are present in the lowest three classes of the total cost of illness. However, 14.3 percent of this category of households is also present in the higher total cost of illness class of above Rs.140000. Three–fourth of the households totally depends on public health centres are there in the lowest two classes of the total cost of illness. It is inferred that households borrowed money for treatment are not only households with informal workers but also households where the income earners are mostly affected.

Table 8.17: Distribution of total cost of illness according to managing the medical expenses

Total cost of illness (in Rs)	Managing the medical expenses					Total
	Past savings	Borrowed money	Friends and relatives	Public health centres	Others	
Less than 2000	38 (39.2)	32 (25.6)	8 (38.1)	5 (62.5)	1 (14.3)	84 (32.6)
2000 - 4000	15 (15.5)	12 (9.6)	4 (19.0)	1 (12.5)	2 (28.6)	34 (13.2)
4000 - 6000	17 (17.5)	15 (12.0)	2 (9.5)	0 (0)	2 (28.6)	36 (14.0)
6000 - 8000	9 (9.3)	21 (16.8)	0 (0)	0 (0)	1 (14.3)	31 (12.0)
8000 - 10000	5 (5.2)	16 (12.8)	3 (0)	0 (0)	0 (0)	24 (9.3)
10000 - 12000	1 (1.0)	4 (3.2)	0 (0)	1 (12.5)	0 (0)	6 (2.3)
12000 - 14000	0 (0)	8 (6.4)	1 (4.8)	1 (12.5)	0 (0)	10 (3)
Above 14000	12 (12.4)	17 (13.6)	3 (14.3)	0 (0)	1 (14.3)	33 (12.8)
Total	97 (100)	125 (100)	21 (100)	8 (100)	7 (100)	258 (100)

Note: Figures in the parentheses show column percentages

18. Experience of Complication

Table 8.18 shows the distribution of the total cost of illness of households according to the category of households experienced complications.

Table 8.18: Total cost of illness according to households experience of complication

Total cost of illness (in Rs)	Experience of complication		Total
	Yes	No	
Less than 2000	15 (27.3)	69 (34.0)	84 (32.6)
2000 - 4000	7 (12.7)	27 (13.3)	34 (13.2)
4000 - 6000	7 (12.7)	29 (14.3)	36 (14.0)
6000 - 8000	5 (9.1)	26 (12.8)	31 (12.0)
8000 - 10000	2 (3.6)	22 (10.8)	24 (9.3)
10000 - 12000	2 (3.6)	4 (2.0)	6 (2.3)
12000 - 14000	2 (3.6)	8 (3.9)	10 (3.9)
Above 14000	15 (27.3)	18 (8.9)	33 (12.8)
Total	55 (100)	203 (100)	258 (100)

Note: Figures in the parentheses show column percentages

The data show that one out of every five households (21.3 percent) experienced complication from the treatment or side effects. Among them 27.3 percent each present in the lowest and highest classes of the total cost of illness, while 74.4 percent of the households not experienced complications are found in the bottom four classes of the total cost of illness. One of the important short – run effects of Chikungunya fever is that the sick persons cannot be able to perform the same work load after the recovery from fever for many days. The information of such households is elicited and the results are shown in Table 8.19.

**Table 8.19: Total cost of illness according to the sick
persons taking the same work load as before**

Total cost of illness (in Rs)	Doing the same work load as before (households)		Total
	Yes	No	
Less than 2000	45 (43.3)	39 (25.3)	84 (25.3)
2000 - 4000	13 (12.5)	21 (13.6)	34 (13.2)
4000 - 6000	17 (16.3)	19 (12.3)	36 (14.0)
6000 - 8000	10 (9.6)	21 (13.6)	31 (12.0)
8000 - 10000	8 (7.7)	16 (10.4)	24 (9.3)
10000 - 12000	2 (1.9)	4 (2.6)	6 (2.3)
12000 - 14000	0 (0)	10 (6.5)	10 (3.9)
Above 14000	9 (8.7)	24 (15.6)	33 (12.8)
Total	104 (100)	154 (100)	258 (100)

Note: Figures in the parentheses show column percentages

It is surprised to note that 59.7 percent (154 out of 258) of the households
have one or more sick persons in the category of not able to take the same
work load when compared to their work performance prior to the infection
of the fever. They are represented in larger percentages in all the classes
except in the bottom two classes of the total cost of illness. However, 43.3
percent of the households reported no change in the work performance
after the infection of Chikungunya fever are represented in the lowest total
cost of illness class. Hence it is clear that the households where the work
performance of the sick members affected have more total cost of illness
when compared to those households where the productively of members not
affected.

19. Type of Patients

Table 8.20 presents the distribution of cost of illness of households
according to the type of patients.

**Table 8.20: Total cost of illness according
to the type of patients**

Total cost of illness	Type of patient-household wise			Total
(in Rs)	Inpatient	Outpatient	Both	
Less than 2000	2 (8.3)	74 (42.0)	4 (7.4)	80 (31.5)
2000 - 4000	5 (20.8)	21 (11.9)	8 (14.8)	34 (13.4)
4000 - 6000	5 (20.8)	21 (11.9)	10 (18.5)	36 (14.2)
6000 - 8000	3 (12.5)	23 (13.1)	5 (9.3)	31 (12.2)
8000 - 10000	4 (16.7)	12 (6.8)	8 (14.8)	24 (9.4)
10000 - 12000	1 (4.2)	5 (2.8)	0 (0)	6 (2.4)
12000 - 14000	2 (8.3)	3 (1.7)	5 (9.3)	10 (3.9)
Above 14000	2 (8.3)	17 (9.7)	14 (25.9)	33 (13.0)
Total	24 (100)	176 (100)	54 (100)	254 (100)

Note: Figures in the parentheses show column percentages

It is found that 68.2 percent of the households have sick members in the category of outpatients. Out of them 42 percent households are found in the lowest total cost of illness class of less than Rs.2000. Among the households having both inpatients and outpatients, 25.9 percent of such households represent the largest total cost of illness class of above Rs.14000. But 70.8 percent of the inpatients are in the lower four classes of total cost of illness from Rs.2000 – 4000 to 8000-10000. It is inferred that households having the category of both inpatients and outpatients have higher total cost of illness followed by inpatients and it is the least in the cases of outpatient households.

20. After-effects of Chikungunya

In Table 8.21 the total cost of illness of households are distributed according to the category of households with after effects.

Table 8.21: Total cost of illness according to the after-effects of Chikungunya

Total cost of illness (in Rs)	After-effects in Households		Total
	Yes	No	
Less than 2000	45 (28.0)	39 (40.2)	84 (32.6)
2000 - 4000	13 (8.1)	21 (21.6)	34 (13.2)
4000 - 6000	21 (13.0)	15 (15.5)	36 (14.0)
6000 - 8000	24 (14.9)	7 (7.2)	31 (12.0)
8000 - 10000	17 (10.6)	7 (7.2)	24 (9.3)
10000 - 12000	3 (1.9)	3 (3.1)	6 (2.3)
12000 - 14000	9 (5.6)	1 (1.0)	10 (3.9)
Above 14000	29 (18.0)	4 (4.1)	33 (12.8)
Total	161 (100)	97 (100)	258 (100)

Note: Figures in the parentheses show column percentages

It is found that 37.6 percent households have no members reported after-effects of Chikungunya fever. Among them 40.2 percent are placed in the lowest total cost of illness class. Moreover 77.3 percent of these households are in the lowest three classes of total cost of illness. It is surprising to note that 62.4 percent households have members with after effects, 23.6 percent are placed in the highest two classes of total cost of illness. Moreover, a majority of such households are concentrated in the middle and upper classes of total cost of illness. It is inferred that the total cost of illness of the households having after-effects is more when compared to the households having no members with after-effects.

Testing of the Hypothesis 1

Null hypothesis: (Ho)

Wage loss to the sick person do not primarily determine the total cost of illness of the Chikungunya affected households

Alternative Hypothesis: (Ha)

Wage loss to the sick person primarily determine the total cost of illness of the Chikungunya affected households

Since the total cost of illness of Chikungunya fever at the household level is a continuous variable, the multidimensionality of total cost of illness is regressed by using the Ordinary Least Square method (OLS). The criterion variable is the total cost illness of households regressed on various predictor variables. The predictor variables consist of many socio-economic and health related variables. Age of the respondent, educational standard of the respondents, monthly household income, suffering period of illness, type of patient, wage loss of the sick person during the period of sickness, wage loss due to side- effects and total numbers of doctor's visit are the predictor variables for the regression analysis. Thus 8 variables have been taken as predictor variables and total cost of illness of the households is the criterion variable. In order to assess the interdependence of the predictor variables, they are subjected to Peterson's Product Moment Correlation Analysis. The computation of the correlation of 8 predictor variables resulted in a correlation matrix; the inter correlation matrix does not show any high degree of correlation between the predictor variables.

In order to find the degree of association between the total cost of illness as the criterion variable and 8 predictor variables given above assume a linear relationship. Household total cost of illness due to Chikungunya fever and its linear relationship with the predictor variables can be expressed as follows.

The functional form can be expressed as follows:

COI=f (AGE, ESTD, TMHINC, SPILL, TYPT, WLDILL, WLDSE, NDOCN)

Where

COI	=	Cost of illness
AGE	=	Age of the head of the household
ESTD	=	Educational standard of the head of the household
TMHINC	=	Total monthly income of the household
SPILL	=	Suffering period of illness
TYPT	=	Type of patient
WLDIE	=	Wage loss due to said effect
NDOCV	=	Number of doctors visit

The estimation of regression equation is done by using step-wise method. The predictor variable is accepted in keeping with the theoretical specification of the regression equation. Moreover, the step-wise regression method has been carried out for the estimation of coefficients for the predictor variables and this has also minimized the problem of multicollinearity. The econometric specification of the final regression model is of the following form:

$$COI = ß_0 + ß_1 AGE + ß_2\ ESTDTM\ ß_3 TMHINC + ß_4 SPILL + ß_5 TYPT + ß_6 WLDILL + ß_7 WLDSE + ß_8 NDOCV + U$$

Where $ß_0$ is constant, $ß_1$ to $ß_8$ are the regression coefficients and U is the error term.

With this econometric specification in the background, the criterion variable and the predictor variables are subjected to the step- wise liner regression. The results have shown that out of the eight predictor variables, the most significant predictor variable is identified in each step. Thus the most significant predictor variable is found in the first step, the second significant in the next step and so on. The present regression model has four steps and that means four significant predictor variables are identified among the eight entered predictor variables. The variable entered and the method adopted is shown in Table 8.22.

Table 8.22: Variables entered and method adopted

Model	Variables Entered	Method
1	Wage loss to the sick person	Stepwise (Criteria: Probability-of-F-to-enter <= .050, Probability-of-F-to-remove >= .100).
2	Wage loss due to side effect	Stepwise (Criteria: Probability-of-F-to-enter <= .050, Probability-of-F-to-remove >= .100).
3	Total number of doctor visits	Stepwise (Criteria: Probability-of-F-to-enter <= .050, Probability-of-F-to-remove >= .100).
4	Type of patient	Stepwise (Criteria: Probability-of-F-to-enter <= .050, Probability-of-F-to-remove >= .100).

The summary results are shown in Table 8.23

Table 8.23: Summary results

Model	R	R Square	Adjusted R Square	Change Statistics		
				R square change	F Change	Sig. F Change
1	.756(a)	.572	.568	.572	149.578	.000
2	.789(b)	.622	.615	.050	14.822	.000
3	.811(c)	.657	.648	.035	11.123	.001
4	.820(d)	.673	.661	.016	5.412	.022

A. Predictors: (Constant), wage loss to the sick person
B. Predictors: (Constant), wage loss to the sick person, Wage loss due to side effect
C. Predictors: (Constant), wage loss to the sick person, Wage loss due to side effect, total number of doctor visits
D. Predictors: (Constant), wage loss to the sick person, Wage loss due to side effect, total number of doctor visits, type of patient

The summery results indicate that wage loss to the sick person is the most significant variable identified because of the high multiple r (R=0.756) which is the correlation between wage loss to the sick person (predictor) and the total cost of illness (criterion). The R^2 value of 0.572 indicates the proportion of the variability in the predictor variable. The second step selected the next important predictor variable (wage loss due to the side-effect) both these variables constitute 62.2 percent of the variability of the criterion variable. Total number of doctor's visits and the type of the patients are the variables identified in the third and fourth steps. All the four variables include in the fourth step of the regression model show that R^2 value of 0.673 All the four predictor variables have fairly high F Change value. The high F change values and the significance of F change value of zero or close to zero shows the strength of the predictor variables. The significant predictor variables in the order of descending importance are wage loss to the sick person, wage loss due to side effect, total number of doctor visits, and type of patient.

Table 8.24: Analysis of variance

Model		Sum of Squares	F	Sig.
1	Regression	4763396163.499	149.578	.000(a)
	Residual	3566697608.791		
	Total	8330093772.289		
2	Regression	5183546150.058	91.429	.000(b)
	Residual	3146547622.231		
	Total	8330093772.289		
3	Regression	5472491615.262	70.219	.000(c)
	Residual	2857602157.027		
	Total	8330093772.289		
4	Regression	5607666541.288	56.130	.000(d)
	Residual	2722427231.001		
	Total	8330093772.289		

The coefficient values of the significantly turned out predictor variables in different steps is shown in Table 8. 25.

Table 8.25: Coefficients

Model	Steps	Unstandardised Coefficients		Standardised Coefficients	t	Sig.
		B	Std.Error	Beta		
1	(Constant)	5874.28	708.020		8.297	.000
	Wage loss to the sick person	1.422	.116	.756	12.230	.000
2	(Constant)	6292.84	676.791		9.298	.000
	Wage loss to the sick person	1.092	.139	.580	7.836	.000
	Wage loss due to side effects	.152	.040	.285	3.850	.000
3	(Constant)	4770.93	792.470		6.020	.000
	Wage loss to the sick person	1.094	.133	.582	8.201	.000
	Wage loss due to side effects	.143	.038	.269	3.778	.000

	Total number of doctor's visits	331.374	99.361	.187	3.335	.001
4	(Constant)	667.733	1927.340		.346	.730
	Wage loss to the sick person	1.099	.131	.584	8.404	.000
	Wage loss due to side effect	.142	.037	.266	3.818	.000
	Total number of doctor visits	351.960	97.827	.199	3.598	.000
	Type of patient	1834.92	788.743	.128	2.326	.022

The coefficients of the excluded variables are shown in Table 8. 26.

Table 8.26: Excluded variables

Model		Beta	t	Sig.	Partial Correlation	Tolerance
1	Age of the respondent	-.033(a)	-.538	.592	-.051	.998
	Educational standard	-.141(a)	-2.198	.030	-.204	.900
	Monthly household income	-.082(a)	-1.327	.187	-.125	.984
	Suffering period of illness	.040(a)	.650	.517	.062	.991
	Type of patient	.112(a)	1.830	.070	.171	1.000
	Wage-loss (side-effect)	.285(a)	3.850	.000	.343	.620
	Number of doctor visits	.202(a)	3.410	.001	.308	.998
2	Age of the respondent	-.010(b)	-.171	.865	-.016	.987
	Educational standard	-.118(b)	-1.937	.055	-.182	.891
	Monthly household income	-.096(b)	-1.638	.104	-.154	.980
	Suffering period of illness	.042(b)	.717	.475	.068	.991
	Type of patient	.110(b)	1.908	.059	.179	1.000

	Number of doctor visits	.187(b)	3.335	.001	.303	.993
3	Age of the respondent	-.006(c)	-.104	.917	-.010	.987
	Educational standard	-.090(c)	-1.512	.133	-.143	.870
	Monthly household income	-.086(c)	-1.530	.129	-.145	.978
	Suffering period of illness	.013(c)	.227	.821	.022	.967
	Type of patient	.128(c)	2.326	.022	.217	.992
4	Age of the respondent	-.011(d)	-.204	.839	-.020	.985
	Educational standard	-.080(d)	-1.357	.178	-.129	.864
	Monthly household income	-.095(d)	-1.725	.087	-.164	.973
	Suffering period of illness	.015(d)	.275	.784	.026	.966

The result of analysis of variance given in Table 8.24 shows that the sum of sequence explained by the regression equation is much higher than the residual sum of squares unexplored. The F value is significant at zero percent level of significance which is well below the probability value of 0.05. From this it is very clear that R^2 value is significantly different from zero in all the four steps. Hence it is correct to assume a linear relationships between the criterion and the four predictor variables and it allows to predict the dependent variable at greater than chance level.

Table 8.25 presents that the high ß values and t values of the predictor variables are significantly different from zero indicate that wage loss to the sick person, wage loss due to side effects, number of doctors visits, and type of patients are the four predictor variables turned out important in the descending order since wage loss to side effects explains 62.2 percent of every Rs.100 increase in the cost of illness of Chikungunya. Hence the analysis accepts the alternative hypothesis and repeals the null hypothesis.

Testing of the Hypothesis 2

Null Hypothesis: (Ho)

Socio-economic, housing and environmental factors are not likely to act more favourably to the infection of Chikungunya fever among wage earner households than non –wage earner households.

Alternative Hypothesis: (Ha)

Socio-economic, housing and environmental factors are likely to act more favourably to the infection of Chikungunya fever among wage earner households than non –wage earner households.

When the dependent variable is not a continuous function, a binary choice model can be assumed when there is a choice between two alternatives and this choice depends on various characteristics of the household. The most commonly used model in such a situation is the logit model.

The logit model estimates the probability of a certain event occurring, given to the set of independent variables. It is based on the probability function and is specified as:

$$P; = F\ (Yi) = f\ (a+bXi) = 1/1+\exp\{-a(a + bxi)\}$$

Where 'exp' is the base of natural logarithms, and Pi is the probability of the occurrence of a certain choice, given the information of Xi. In this model, the dependent variable is the probability that a wage earner household is affected by the Chikungunya fever. The left hand side of the logit model is easy to predict the effect of change of any of the explanatory variable on the probability of the observation belonging to other wage earner affected or not affected in a household.

The logit model has sixteen independent variables in the function of wage earners affected due to Chikungunya in a household. They are:

AGE	=	Age of the head of the house hold
EDUSTD	=	Educational standard of the head of the household
HSIZE	=	Household size
TMHINCOM	=	Total Monthly Household Income

TENNAT   =   Nature of Tenancy
HOEELECT   =   Electrification of the House
DVEHRES   =   Distance between Residence and Vehicular Path
WATSTAG   =   Water Stagnation
WATSTOE   =   Water Storing Mechanism
OPENAREA   =   Availability of Open Area
BANAPLAN   =   Availability of Banana Plantations
ROBBRPLA   =   Availability of Rubber plantations
TOILET   =   Availability of Toilet
REARCA   =   Rearing of Animals
NOCHICKA   =   No. of Members Affected by Chikungunya
TESTFEE   =   Fees paid for testing

Among the independent variables, the following subjective variables are used by dummy values:

Educational Status: 0 = Illiterate, 1 = Primary, 2 = Middle, 3 = High, 4=High second/PUC, 5 = Bachelor's Degree, 6 = Masters, 7 = Professionals, 8 = Highly Educated.

TENNAT: 1 = owned, 2 = Leased, 3 = Rented.
Electrification of House: Yes = 1, No= 0
Water Stagnation: Yes = 1, No = 0
Water Storing Mechanism: Yes = 1, No = 0
Availability of Open Area: Yes = 1, No = 0
Availability of Banana Plantations: Yes = 1, No = 0
Availability of Rubber Plantations: Yes = 1, No = 0
Availability of Toilet: Yes =1, No = 0
Rearing of Animals: Yes = 1, No = 0

The actual values are taken for the continuous variables such as the age of the head of the household, household size, total monthly household income, distance between residence and the vehicular road, total number of members affected by Chikungunya fever and total test fees. In the logistic regression model, in order to interpret the coefficients, the model can be re written in terms of the odds ratio of the event occurring, which is defined as the ratio of probability occurrence of an event to the probability that it does not occur. (Pi/ 1-Pi). The results are given in Table 8.27.

Table 8.27: Dependent variable encoding

Original Value	Internal Value
No	0
Yes	1

It shows that the dependant variable is the wage earners affected households. It is a binary variable. 'Yes' is denoted by the value '1' and 'No' is denoted by '0'. Thus positive coefficient indicates that an increasing value of that variable involves an increasing likelihood of a favourable response. The classifications are furnished in Table 8.28.

Table 8.28: Classification Table

	Observed		Predicted		
			Wage earners affected		Percentage Correct
Step 0			No	Yes	
	Wage earners affected	No	0	38	.0
		Yes	0	92	100.0
	Overall Percentage				70.8

It helps to assess the performance of the model by cross tabulating the observed response categories. The predicted category is treated as 1, if that category's predicted value is greater than the cut off. The variables in the equation are shown in Table 8.29.

In the Zero Blocks, NOCHICKA, EDUSTO TESTFEE, ROBBRPLA, BANALAN, WATSTOE and WATSTGA are considered significant because of their high score and lowest P value.

Table 8.29: Variables in the equation

			Score	Degrees of freedom	Sig.
Step 0	Variables	AGE	.047	1	.829
		EDUSTD	5.192	1	.023
		HSIZE	.904	1	.342
		TMHINCOM	.734	1	.392
		TENNAT	.839	1	.360
		HOEELECT	.292	1	.589
		DVEHPRES	.407	1	.524
		WATSTGA	1.339	1	.247
		WATSTOE	1.477	1	.224
		OPENAREA	.165	1	.685
		BANAPLAN	1.197	1	.274
		ROBBRPLA	3.507	1	.061
		TOILET	.000	1	.995
		REARCP	.299	1	.585
		NOCHICKA	15.852	1	.000
		TESTFEE	4.437	1	.035

The model summary is given in Table 8.30.

Table 8.30: Model Summary

Step	-2 Log likelihood	Cox & Snell R Square	Nagelkerke R Square
1	106.656	.322	.459

The 2 – log likelihood and Psedo R^2 statistics computed at each step in the model, R^2 value of Cox and Snell appears 0.322 and Nagelkerke R Square is found as 0.459. It shows that the environmental and the housing variables have more influence on the infection of Chikungunya to a wage earner in a household than a non wage earner.

The variables in the equation is given in Table 8.31

Table 8.31: Variables in the equation

		B	S.E.	Wald	Degrees of freedom	Sig.	Exp(B)
Step 1(a)	AGE	-.014	.021	.479	1	.489	.986
	EDUSTD	-.183	.180	1.033	1	.309	.833
	HSIZE	.092	.234	.154	1	.695	1.096
	TMHINCOM	.000	.000	3.567	1	.059	1.000
	TENNAT	17.359	27617.246	.000	1	.999	34600090.585
	HOEELECT	1.877	1.648	1.297	1	.255	6.532
	DVEHPRES	.000	.000	.052	1	.819	1.000
	WATSTGA	.772	.593	1.694	1	.193	2.164
	WATSTOE	-.568	.486	1.366	1	.243	.567
	OPENAREA	.155	.545	.081	1	.776	1.168
	BANAPLAN	.003	.679	.000	1	.996	1.003
	ROBBRPLA	-2.170	.662	10.733	1	.001	.114
	TOILET	-.615	.658	.872	1	.350	.541
	REARCP	.378	.581	.423	1	.515	1.460
	NOCHICKA	2.707	.741	13.338	1	.000	14.980
	TESTFEE	.001	.001	3.877	1	.049	1.001
	Constant	-18.614	27617.246	.000	1	.999	.000

According to the values of Wald Statistics TENNAT, BANAPLA, AGE, DVEHPRES and OPEWAR show the significant results. EXP (B) is in favour in the case of NOCHICKA, HOEELECT, WATSGA, TENNAT, OPENAR, and BANAPLAN. These variables have significant odds ratio. The result show that the important factors determining the infection of Chikungunya to wage earning households are:

The fitted logistic model:

$$\pi_x = \frac{exp\,(-18.614-0.014X1-183X2+0.092X3+0.00X4+17.359X5+1.877X6}{1+exp(-18.614-0.014X_1-183X_2+0.092X_3+.00x4X_4+17.359X_5+1.877X_6}$$

$$+\;0.00X_7+0.772X_8-0.568X_9+0.155X_{10}+0.03X_{11}-2.170X_{12}-0.615X_{13}+$$
$$+\;0.000X_7+0.772X_9-0.586X_9+0.155X_{10}+0.03X_{11}-2.170X_{12}-0.615X_{13+}$$
$$0.378X_{11}+2.707X_{15}+0.001X_{16}$$
$$0.378X_{14}+2.707X_{15}+0.001X_{16}.$$

Where in the above equation X_1 to X_{16} are the explanatory variables. These statistics clearly reveal that environmental variables have more probability of infecting the wage earner of a household to Chikungunya fever than a non wage earner.

The analysis vividly makes the point clear that infection of communicable diseases to the workforce in the informal sector impact the household budget severely at least in the short run. Chikungunya infection is a kind of epidemic causing inability to perform the regular work after the recovery for months together. The disease was not given the due importance on the hope that it is not fatal. The economic loss of the households of the poor sections of the society with employed members affected forced them to perennial indebtedness.

Summary Of The Findings And Suggestions

C hikungunya is an infectious disease caused by mosquitoes. The recent attack in many parts of the country had debilitating infection in working population heralded by fever, anthralgia, rash, pain and swellings that not only did not allow the patients to perform their daily tasks but also difficult for them to regain their ability to resume work. Though Chikungunya fever is not fatal, it caused severe hardships to the households socially, economically and medically by having severe morbidity and disability. These factors have adversely affected the household production function and negative spill -over effects at the national level.

The present study made sincere attempt to analyse the economic burden of the Chikungunya affected households in Vilavancode and Kalkulam Taluk of Kanyakumari District of Tamil Nadu. The data necessary for the analysis have been collected from 258 sample households. Kanyakumari is one of the smallest districts of Tamil Nadu having agriculture as the main occupation which include Rubber, coconut, banana and spice plantations besides vegetable and paddy fields. The district has the peculiar distinction of getting rainfall both during South-West and North-East monsoons. The climate conditions and agricultural pattern are conducive for the breeding of mosquitoes.

Every one of five sample households is headed by women. Out of the total households 57 percent are headed by persons aged between 25 and 50 years of age and around 40 percent between 50 and 75 years of age. Married respondents account for 89.9 percent. More than one-third have high school level education and 77.3 percent have education not above the school level. Hence the Chikungunya affected households are headed by people having lesser level of education. Around half of the total respondents are engaged as unskilled labourers. The educational pattern of the respondents reflects that most of the respondents have only school level education in a district where the level of education is the highest level in Tamil Nadu.

Among the total households, 74 percent belong to the Nadar community comprising 49.2 and 24.8 percentages respectively of Christian Nadars and

Hindu Nadars. Backward class households form 77.1 percent, followed by Scheduled Caste and others in the proportion of 7.8 and 11.2 percentages respectively. It is found that 60.5 percent of the households are Christians and 83.7 percent speak Tamil. Nuclear families are predominant comprising 86.4 percent. The average size of the household is 3.9 comprising 1.27 male members and 1.24 female members. The average size of female members (1.63) appears slightly bigger that of the same of male members (1.55). However, employed male member households are almost four times that of the same of households with female employed. The average male member employed in a household is worked as 1.30 as compared to 1.31 of the average female members employed. The percentage share of households with illiterate members accounts for 23.26 percent.

Out of the 258 households, 92.25 percent have at least one male income earner when compared to 24.03 households with at least one female earner. The average income of the head of the households is higher than the average income of family members. The average monthly income of the sample household is computed as Rs.12264. More than half of the total number of households earns a monthly income less than Rs.7500. Every four out of five households (88.37 percent) have members taking food outside home. The average monthly income of food taken outside is Rs.526.91 and average monthly household expenditure on food is computed as Rs.2838.45 that is 23.14 percentage of the average monthly household income. It is noteworthy that debt repayment occupies the second largest expenditure. More than two-fifth (42.6 percent) incur an average household monthly expenditure between Rs.4000 – Rs.6000. Out of the total sample households 56.2 percent affirmed having some form of savings and the average household savings is Rs.17,976. Out of them 33.1 percent is found in the lowest class of savings of less than Rs.3000 and 20 percent in the highest savings class of Rs.18000 and above. It is found that 71.3 percent of the households are debtors and 55.4 percent of them have a debt of less than Rs.50000. Indebtedness is deep-rooted among majority of the sample households. The average possession of wealth by the households is valued at Rs. 8.27 lakhs.

It is important to note that 96.1 percent of the households own their residence and 96.1 percent of the houses are electrified. The average housing area of sample households is 784.74 sq.ft. More than half (55.8 percent) of the households possess houses with concrete roof. The average number of windows and rooms are 5.14 and 3.2 respectively. Nearly half of the households have vehicular road as the access way to their houses.

The average distance between residence and vehicular road is estimated at 495.08 metres.

Nearly half (49.6 percent) of the residences are located near water stagnating area. Most of the residences except those situated adjacent to the vehicular roads are isolated and hence used to have open area near their residences. Nearly half (46.9 percent) of the households have open-well for the drinking purpose and public tap for drinking water accounts 40.3 percent. Pots and overhead tank are the two important water storing mechanism accounting for 47.7 and 43.8 percentages respectively. It is found that 44.6 percent of the household dispose waste in their backyards and disposal site as the disposing area for 45 percent of the households. The presence of open area, banana plantations and rubber plantations are for 52.3, 70.2 and 61.6 percentages of the households respectively. More than two-thirds of the households (68.6 percent) have separate closed toilet facilities. It is reported that 27.5 percent households rear cattle and pet animals in their vicinity.

The average number of households affected by Chikungunya fever is 1.56. Children and aged members infected by Chikungunya fever account for 7.36 and 16.28 percentages respectively of the sample households. The literatures have shown that in many of the States children and aged members are common among the victims of Chikungunya fever. The average number of male children affected is 1.1 as compared to 1.0 of female children. The members affected in the working age group comprise 86.05 percent of the sample households. The average number of male and female members affected is 1.07 and 1.4 respectively. It is found that 61.2 percent of the sample households have a single member affected by the Chikungunya fever. Households with two, three, four and five members affected are in the percentages of 25.2, 10.1, 3.1 and 0.4 respectively. Among the male and female children affected households, 89.5 and 100 percentages respectively have a single child affected.

Among the households having male working aged members affected, 93.7 percent have a single member affected. It is 88.2 percent in the case of households having number of female members affected. Households with single member affected among the households having working aged population affected account for 64.4 percent. Households with two, three and four members affected in the working age population comprise 26.6, 6.8 and 2.3 percentages respectively. The pattern of infection of Chikungunya fever revealed that even though 63.6 percent of the households having a single member affected 21.7 percent households come under the category of some members affected simultaneously and some members affected in different periods in a year account for 3.9 and 1.9 percentages respectively.

It is reported that 71.3 percent of the households have identified the fever as Chikungunya after doctor's diagnosis, however clinical examination and clinical symptoms as methods of identification in the case of 13.34 and 18.6 percentages respectively. More than two-thirds (64.7 percent) of the sample households have at least one member affected due to Chikungunya fever. More than four-fifth (83.8 percent) of the wage earner affected households have a single wage earner affected by the fever. Nearly half (48.4 percent) of the sample households borrowed money to meet the medical expenditure and 37.6 percent used their past savings for this purpose. Out of the 248 households 94.96 percent treated the pain of the fever is severe followed by moderate pain and mild pain accounting for 6.2 and 1.6 percentages respectively.

All the sample households expressed that sudden fever was the initial symptom. Joint pain was the second most important symptom accounting 98.45 percent of the households. Other symptoms in the order of importance were cough and headache. Rash and swellings were accounted by 43.35 percent of the households. Among the different symptoms joint pain and swelling continued for a long period of time. Nearly two-thirds of the households reported the problem of side effects or aftermath effect after the recovery of Chikungunya fever. It is found that 57.3 percent of the households having married members have a single member affected, while it is 84.8 percent in the case of unmarried member affected households. No household has more than two unmarried members affected by the Chikungunya fever. Around 80 percent of the sample households depended on private medical practitioners for medical assistance. As such as 17.2 percent households fully depended on public medical facilities, while 3.5 percent utilised both private and public medical care facilities.

Allopathy is the type of medical treatment practised by 95.74 percent of the households having 1.4 sick persons per household. Homeopathy, Ayurvedic and Sidha ways of treatment account for 2.71, 1.94 and 1.63 percentages respectively of the total households. Diabetes is the most common non-communicable health problem of the sick person affected by Chikungunya fever (18.99 percent). Sleeplessness was the problem expressed by 89.53 percent of the sample households. Households reporting the problem of sleeplessness for single, two, three and four sick persons account for 68.4, 23.4, 6.1, and 2.2 percentages respectively. Only 10.9 percent of the households opined that in their households Chikungunya fever repeated more than once. But none gave the information that the fever repeated in the same person more than once. It is found that 98.1 percent of the households consulted doctor for treating Chikungunya fever. More than 20 percent of the households reported complication of treatment. It is found that 75.97 percent of the households had taken the patient to the doctor as soon as they felt the symptoms of Chikungunya fever.

The average duration of recovery from the disease is 13.12 days and the average time taken for normalcy and suffering period of the disease are 50.97 days and 190.25 days respectively. Three–fifth (59.7 percent) of the households having members affected could not carry the same workload previous to the infection of the fever. But only 22.1 percent of the households accepted having members changed their occupation after the infection of Chikungunya fever.

The category of patients as outpatients, outpatients and inpatients and inpatients are in the percentages of 69.3, 21.3 and 9.4 respectively. Out of 253 households consulted doctors, 47.4 percent made a single visit. Households made 2-4 visits account for 24.1 percent.

The estimation of the direct cost of illness of the outpatients, the average doctor's fee, cost of medicines, cost of tests and transportation cost are Rs.753.5, Rs.1059.85 and Rs.422.19 and Rs.207.42 respectively. The cost components of cost of illness of inpatients such as doctor's fee, diagnostic tests, and accommodation and transportation costs account for Rs. 642.5, Rs.674, Rs.1796.82 and Rs. 273.57 respectively. The analysis has taken wage loss as the only indirect cost. The wage losses to the sick person, caretaker and wage loss due to the side effects are Rs.3448.66, Rs. 1691.3 and Rs. 5863.93 respectively. The average wage loss due to side effects is the highest and it is almost twice as that of the wage loss of the sick persons during the sick period. The wage loss to the caretakers is relatively not substantial.

It is found that the total cost of illness is less than Rs. 2000 for nearly one-third (32.6 percent) of the sample households. The next largest proportion of 14 percent households represents the expenditure class of Rs.4000 – Rs. 6000. The average cost of illness of the sample households is calculated as Rs. 6658.31.

The comparison of the COI of households with age of the head of the households revealed that more than two-thirds of the young respondents and 80 percent of the respondents above 75 years are found in the lowest total cost of illness class of less than Rs.2000. Around 50 percent of the households of the respondents aged between 25 and 50 years are found in the higher cost of illness classes of Rs. 6000 and above.

With regard to the distribution of COI according to the gender of the respondents, more percentage share of the households of the women respondents are found in the lowest two COI classes. In the higher COI classes expect Rs.6000 – Rs.8000 and Rs.10000 – Rs.12000 the male headed households have more representation. With regard to the distribution of COI according to communities, the Backward Class households are the least in the lowest class of total COI accounting 29.1 percent as compared to the highest of 62.5 percent by Most Backward Class households. The Backward Class households have more representation in the highest class total COI. Among the different religions, Hindus share 23.3 percent in the higher total COI as compared to 16.6 percent of the Christians. Moreover 65.7 percent of the households headed by illiterate persons are in the total COI classes of less than Rs. 4000. The general trend is that the literate respondents headed households spent relatively more for defending the sickness. Among the literate households, 60 percent of the households headed by graduates and 100 percent of the post graduate households are placed in the lowest class of total COI. The households of school level educated heads are found in all classes of total cost of illness.

Nearly three –fifth of the joint families (58.1 percent) represent the lowest total COI classes of less than Rs.4000 as compared to 43 percent of the same of the nuclear families.Most of the employees of the formal sector are concentrated in the lowest class of total COI because absence of work during the sick period and the period of side effects has less impact on their income generation. Most of the employees get wages during the period of absence from work due to the sickness. Informal workers are among the sick persons in 93.8 percent of the sample households. Households of the sick persons engaged in informal occupations are the worst affected because their work involve more physical strength, no payment for the days of unemployment and the after effects are comparatively for a prolonged period. These issues worked in favour of their indebtedness.

The comparison between size of the household and total COI has shown that 41.7 percent of the households with two members are found in the lowest cost of illness class. The highest total COI classes of Rs. 14000 and above comprise households having a size between two and five, i.e., 17.1 percent households with four members and 8.2 percent with five members. However, households with a higher household size of six, seven and eight consists of

100.0, 70.0 and 66.7 percentages respectively in the lower three classes of the total COI.

The distribution of total COI across different income groups has revealed that 55.5 percent of the lowest income households are found in the lowest class of total COI. In all the income classes except Rs. 8000 – Rs.10000 and Rs.10000–12000, maximum percentage share of households present in the total COI class of less than Rs.2000. In the highest total COI class of Rs. 14000 and above 27.7 percent of the households having a monthly income of Rs.7501 to Rs.10000 are present. Though high income households have relatively higher percentage share in the highest total COI class, households in the higher income groups of Rs.12501–Rs.15000 and Rs.15001–Rs.17000 consists of 66.8 and 60.8 percentages respectively present in the lowest two classes of total COI. This paradox is due to the fact that the high income households are mostly literate who had the knowledge of non-fatality of the disease, non-availability of medicines and the need for rest and the use of mild pain killer to relieve the pain. However poor households are mostly illiterate or having lesser educational standard become panic about the fever and feeling similar to Malaria or Dengue, hence treated the disease at a high costs, even by borrowing money at high rate of interest.

Out of 71.32 percent of the indebted households 31.5 percent are in the lowest total COI. In the highest total COI class, the indebted households account for 15.2 percent. Among, the highest level of indebted class of Rs. 2 lakh and above, 43.8 percent belong to the class of the lowest total COI of less than Rs.2000. It is observed and the data strongly support that most of the households in lower indebted classes borrowed money for meeting medical expenditure and the expenses related to the unemployment due to sickness. However, households in the higher indebted classes either borrowed money for any non-medical expenditure or part of the debt is meant for defending the disease.

The distribution cost of illness across households in different sizes of houses presents that more than 50 percent of the households lived in largest houses of above 1000 sq.ft are in the lowest level of total COI, while only 19.7 percent of the households in house size less than 500 sq.ft are the lowest COI class. The relationship emerged is that the households lived in bigger sized houses are found in the lower cost of illness and vice versa. The percentage share of households who have access way to their houses in the category of vehicular road, paved path and unpaved path in the lower four classes of total COI are 68.8, 74.5 and 76.5 percentages respectively.

It means closer the household to the vehicular path lesser is the total COI. Relatively more households having larger distance from vehicular road is found in the higher classes of total COI.

More than two –fifth (43 percent) of the households with single member affected have the least total COI and 12.7 percent in the highest class of total COI. But most of the households with two and three sick persons are found in the middle classes of total COI. More than half (52.7 percent) of the households having no wage earner affected are placed in the lowest total COI class while 37.8 percent of the wage-earner affected households are in the higher total COI classes of Rs.8000 and more. In general the number of households having no wage earner affected are found less when go up in the total COI, while more percentage share of wage earners affected households are found in higher classes of total cost of illness.

More than one-fourth (25.6 percent) of the households borrowed money to meet the medical expenses are in the lowest COI class of less than Rs.2000 when compared to 39.2 percent of the households who met the medical expenses from their own savings. More than three fifth (62.5 percent) of the households depend public health centres are found in the lowest class of total COI. The survey revealed that one out of every –five households having sick members experienced complication from treatment or side effects. Among them 27.3 percent each present in the lowest and highest classes of the total cost of illness. It is found that 74.4 percent of the households not experienced complications are found in the bottom four classes of total COI. Among the 59.7 percent of the households having members not able to take the same workload are found 38.5 percent in the bottom two classes of COI when compared to 55.8 percentage of the households having members who can take the same workload previous to the infection of the Chikungunya fever.

There are 68.2 percent of the households have sick members in the category of outpatients. Out of them 42 percent are found in the lowest total COI. More than one fourth (25.9 percent) of the household having both inpatients and outpatients category of sick persons are found in the highest total COI class of Rs.14000 and above. It is inferred that households with both inpatients and outpatients have higher total cost of illness followed by inpatients and outpatients households.

The testing of the hypothesis "wage loss to the sick person primarily determine the total cost of illness of the Chikungunya affected households" by apply stepwise multiple regression model has shown that the most significant variables in the four steps are wage loss to the sick person, wage loss due to the side effect total number of doctor's visit and type of patients. All the four variables in the model had shown the R^2 value of 0.673. All the four variables have high F change values and the significance close to zero shown the strength of predictor variables. Hence the analysis accepted the alternative hypothesis.

The second hypothesis taken is that the socio-economic, housing and environmental factors are likely to act more favourably to the infection of Chikungunya fever among wage earner households them non-wage earner households. This hypothesis is tested by using logit model. According to the Wald statistics the environmental variables have more predictability of infecting the wage earner households then the non-wage earner household. The results show that environmental variables have high probability of infecting the wage earner than a non wage earner household.

SUGGESTIONS

1. Each district should be set up with a medical emergency unit to address to needs of communicable diseases.
2. Each village Panchayat should take necessary steps to control mosquitoes' periodically.
3. Bio-vector control, pesticide use, awareness creating programmes should be conducted to improve health and hygiene conditions.
4. Vector control programme should consist of a specialist to undertake surveillance and evaluation of control programme.
5. All informal workers must compulsorily be brought under unemployment relief network in the case of disability to perform work after any medical problem.
6. Informal workers should be given paid holidays during the period of hospital admission.
7. All community health centres should be provided with sufficient medical staff and medicines to address infectious diseases.
8. Make it compulsory to keep the coconut shell upside down after the collection of tapped rubber from rubber trees.
9. Banana plantations near domestic area are also the source of mosquito breeding. Take steps to prevent stagnation of water in the cultivation lanes.
10. A Medical Disaster Management team should be trained in each district to attend the epidemics due to infectious diseases.

11. A medical protocol should be immediately circulated among the medical practitioners in the event of a new disease emerging to avoid complications in treatment.

12. Measures need to be worked out to address the exclusion of poor from public health-care facilities.

13. Given the conditions that there is no guarantee of wage during the sick days of the informal workers, replacing the Public Health Facilities with cash payment for wages during the sick days will enable them to take private medical care if warranted.

14. Increased feminisation of informal employment disempower women more during the period of sickness. Since women workers have less bargaining power in household decision making, they get poor or no medical care during the period of sickness. There is a need for sick period relief measures with special reference to informal women workers.

Bibliography

Abel-Smith B, Rawal P, 1994, 'Employer's Willingness to Pay: The Case for Compulsory Health Insurance in Tanzania', *Health Policy and Planning,* 9(4).

Adhikari S.R, Maskay N.M, 2003, 'The Economic Burden of Kalazan in Household of the Danusna and Mahottari Districts of Nepal', *Acta Trop,* 88.

American Diabetes Association, 'Economic Costs of Diabetes in the US in 2002', *Diabetes Care 2003*, 26(3).

Andreano and Helminiak, 1988, 'Economic, Health and Tropical Disease; A Review in Economics', *Health and Tropical Disease*, University of Philippines School of Economics.

Armien B, Suaya JA, Quiroz EQ, San BK, Bayard V, (et al), 2008, 'Clinical Characteristics and National Economics Cost of the 2005 Dengue Epidemic in Panama' *AM J Tropical Medicines and Hygiene,* 73.

Arrow, K.J., H.B. Chenery, B.S. Minhas, and R.M. Solow, 1961, 'Capital-Labor Substitution and Economic Efficiency', *Review of Economic Studies,* 43.

Athreya Venkatesh and Sheela Rani Chunkath, 1998, 'Gender and Infant Survival in Rural Tamil Nadu: Situation and Strategy' *Economic and Political Weekly.*

Bajpai P.K, 1998, *Social work perspective on Health*, Rawat Publishing, New Delhi.

Banerjee K, Mourya D.T, Malunjkar, 1988, 'As Susceptibility and Transmissibility of Different Geographical Strains of Aedes aegypti Mosquitoes to Chikungunya Virus India', *Journal of Medical Research*, 87.

Barger K, Ehlken B, Kugland B, Augustin M, 2005, 'Cost of Illness in Patients with Moderate and Severe Chronic Psoriasis Vulgar in Germany' *J Dtsch Dermatology Ges*, 3.

Barron R, Sala-I-Martin X, 1995, *Economic Growth*, McGraw-Hill, New York.

Bartlett J.C, Miller L.S, Rice D.P, Max W, 1994, 'Medical Care Expenditures Attributable to Cigarette Smoking – United States', *Morbidity Mortality weekly Report,* 43.

Baskara Rao N, 1976 *Family Panning in India,* Vikas Publishing House Private Ltd, New Delhi.

Benenson A. S, 1995, 'Control of Communicable Diseases in Man', 16 Ed., USA, *American Public Health Association.*

Benichou J A, 2001, 'Review of Adjusted Estimators of Attributable Risk', *Statistical Methods in Medical Research,* 10(3).

Berman Peter, 1995, *Health Sector Reform in Developing Countries. Making Health Development Sustainable,* Harvard University Press, Boston.

Berndt, Ernst R, 2007, 'Advance Market Commitments for Vaccines against Neglected Diseases: Estimating Cost and Effectiveness', *Health Economics,* Vol, 16.Issues, 5.

Bhargava A, Jamison D, Lau L, Murray C, 2001, 'Modeling the Effects of Health on Economic Growth', *Journal of Health Economics,* 20.

Bhat Ramesh and Saha Somen, 2004, 'Health Insurance Not a Panacea', *Economic and Political Weekly,* August 14.

Bloom B S, Bruno D J, Maman D y, and Jayadevappa R, 2001 'Usefulness of US Cost of Illness Studies in Healthcare Decision Making, *Pharmacoeconpmics,* 19(2).

Bloom DE, Canning D, 2006, 'Epidemics and Economics, Program on the Global Demography of Aging' *Working Paper No.9,* Harvard initiative for Global Health.

Bloom DE, Canning D, Seville J, 2004, 'The Effect of Health on Economic Growth: A Production Function Approach,' *World Development,* 32.

Bodemman P, Genton B, 2006, 'Chikungunya: An Epidemic in Real Time' *Lancet,* No, 368.

Bodenmann P, Genton B, 2006, 'Chikungunya, 'An Epidemic in Real Time', *Lancet,* 368.

Bose Ashish, Devenora et al, (ed.), 2002, *Social Statistics, Health and Education,* Vikas Publishing House Private Ltd., New Delhi.

Bradlay D.J, 1993, 'Human Tropical Diseases in a Changing Environment', *CIBA Foundation Symposium,* 175:146-62; Discussion.

Bridgman R.F, 1970, *The Rural Hospital; Its Structure and Organization*s, World Health Organisation, Geneva.

Briggs A, 1999, 'Handling Uncertainty in Economic Evaluation' *B M J,* 319(7202).

Brighton S.W, 1981, 'Chikungunya Virus Infections,' *South African Medical Journal*, 59.

Brighton S.W, Prozesky O.W, de la Harpe A.L, 1983, 'Chikungunya Virus Infection A retrospective Study of 107 Cases,' *South African Medical Journal,* 63.

Brignton S.W, Porzesky O.W, Harpe A.L, 1982, 'Chikungunya Virus Infection: A Retrospective Study of 107 Cases,' *South African Medical Journal*, 63.

Broot G.D, 1938, *Health through Project,* Barnes and Company, New York.

Burton I, R. W Kates and G.F. White, 1993, *The Environment as a Hazard*, Guilford Press, New York.

Campos L.E, San Juan A, Cenabre L.C, Alrnagro E.E, 1969, 'Isolation of Chikungunya Virus in the Philippines,' *Acta Med Philipp,* 552(4).

Casman E.A and H. Dowlatabadi, 2002, *Contextual Determinants of Malaria*, Resources for the Future Press, Washington, D C.

Centre for Science and Environment, 2010, *Down to Earth,* 41.

Chalkely A.M, 1986, *A Text Book for the Health workers*, The Christian Literature Society, Madras.

Chan N.Y, Eb K.L, Smith F, Wilson T. F, and, Smith, A.E, 1999, An Integrated Assessment Framework for Climate Change and Infectious Diseases, *Environmental Health Perspectives,* 107.

Chauhan Devraj and Sangita Kamdar, 1997, 'Social Sector and Development Focus on Health Care', *Yojana*, Vol.41, No, 4.

Chow, Jeffrey; Darley, Sarah R; Laxminarayan, Ramananm, 2007, 'Cost-effectiveness of Disease Interventions in India'.

Cll-Mckinsey and Company, 2003, 'Healthcare in India: The Road Ahead', *Ninth Five year Plan: 1997-2002*, Government of India, New Delhi.

Cohen D R and Henderson J B, 1988, 'Health Prevention and economics', Oxford University press.

Colwell R.R, and Patz J, 1998, *A Climate Infections Disease and Health*, American Academy of Microbiology, Washington D C, USA.

Colwell R.R, 1996, 'Global Climate and Infections Disease: The Cholera Paradigm', *Science,* 274 (5295).

Cooper B S and Rice D P, 1976, 'The Economic Cost of Illness Revisited', *Social Security Bulletin*, 39(2).

Cooper Michael H. and Antony (ed.),1973, *Health Economics*, Penguin Books Ltd, England.

Cummings D.A, Irizarry R.A, Huang N.E, Endy T.P, Nisalak A, et al, 2004, 'Travelling Waves in the Occurrence of Dengue Hemorrhagic Fever in Thailand', *Nature*, 427.

Currie G, kerfoot K D, Donaldson C, and Macarthur C, 2006, 'Are Cost of Injury Studies Use full?', *Injury Prevention*, 6.

Dandawate C.N, Thiruvengadam K.V, Kalyansundram V, Rajagopal J, Rao TR, 1965, 'Serological Survey in Madras City with Special reference to Chikungunya', *Indian med res,* 53.

Diallo M, Thonnon J, Traore Laminana M, Fonteille D, 1999, 'Vectors of Chikungunya Virus in Senegal: Current Data and Transmission Cycles', *AMJ Tropical Medicine Hygiene*, 60.

Drummond M, 1992, 'Cost-of-illness Studies; A Major Headache?' *Pharmaco economics*, 2(1).

Drummond. M F,1997, Et al (eds), 'Methods for the Economic Evaluations of Health Care Programmers', 2nd Edition, Oxford University Press.

Enserink.M, 2006, 'Massive Outbreak Draws Fresh Attention to Little Known Virus', *Science*, Vol. 311, No.1085.

Epstein, Paul R, 2006, 'Climate Change and Public Health: Focusing on Emerging Infectious Diseases', *Smart Growth and Climate Change: Regional Development, Infrastructure and Adaptation*.

EpsteinP.R, 1999, 'Climate and health', *Science*, 285.

Finkelstein E.A, Fiebelkorn I.C, and Wang G, 2003, 'National medical spending Attributable to Overweight and obesity: How Much and who's paying', *Health Affairs*, 14 may: 219, w3.

Finkler S A, 1982, 'The Distinction between Costs and Charges', *Annals of Internal Medicine*, 96.

Flegal K M, Graubard B I, Williamson D F, and Gail M H, 2005, 'Excess Deaths Associated with Underweight, Overweight, and Obesity', *JAMA*, 293 (115).

Flegal K M, Graubard B I, and Williamson D F, 2004, 'Methods of Calculating Deaths Attributable to Obesity', *American Journal of Epidemiology*, 160(4).

Ford S, Torgerson D J, Raftery J, 2000, 'Cost of Illness Studies', *BMJ*, 320.

Fradin M.S,Day J.F, 2002, 'Comparative Efficacy of Insect: Repellent Against Mosquito Bites,' *N English Journal of Medicine*, 347.

FRCH, 1987, *Health Status of the Indian People: Supplementary Document to Health for All- An Alternative Strategy,* Foundation for Research in Community Health, Bombay.

Freedberg K A, Scharfstein J A, Seage G R III, L osina E, Weinstein M C, Craven D E, and paltiel A D,1998, 'The Cost-Effectiveness of Preventing AIDS-Related Opportunistic Infections', *JAMA*, 279(2).

French M T and Martin R F, 1996, 'The Costs of Drug Abuse Consequences'-A Summary of Research Findings', *Journal of Substance Abuse Treatment*, 13(6).

Gallup J, Sad us J, 2001, 'The Economic Burden of Malaria', *Am J Trop Med Hyg,* 64 (Suppl).

Ganesan K, Diwan A, Shankar S.K, Desai S.B, Sainani G.S, Kartak S.M, 2008, 'Chikungunya Encephalomyeloradicultis: Report of 2 Cases with Neuroimaging and 1Case with Autopsy Findings', *AJNR American Journal of Neuroradiol.*

Garg P, Nag Pal J, Khairnar P, Seneviratne SL, 2008, 'Economic Burden of Dengue Infections in India', *Trans R Society of Tropical Medicine and Hygiene,* 102.

Gerardin P, Baraurer, Michault A, (et al),2006, 'Multi- disciplinary Prospective Study of Mother-to-Child Transmission of Chikungunya Virus Infections on the Island of La Reunion,' *PLOS Medicine*, Vol.5, No 3 eto doi: 10.1371/ Tournal.pmed.0050060.

Gerpvotz, Mark,Hammer, Jeffrey S, 2004, 'The Economical Control of infectious Diseases,' *Economic Journal*, Vol.114, Issue, 492.

Gersovitz, Mark, 2000, 'A Preface to the Economic Analysis of Disease Transmission', *Australian Economic Papers*, Vol. 39, issue. 1.

Gibbons R.V, Vaughn D.W, 2002, 'Dengue: An Escalating Problem', *Bangladesh Medical Journal*, 324.

Goetzel R. Z, Long S.R, Ozminkowski R.J, Hawkins K, Wang S, Lynch W, 2004, 'Health Absence, Disability, and Presenteeism Cost Estimates of Certain Physical and Mental Health Conditions Affecting U S Employers'. *Journal of Occupational and Environmental Medicine*, 46.

Gold M R, Siegel J E, Russell L B, and Weinstein M C, 1996, 'Cost Effectiveness in Health and Medicine', Oxford University Press, New York.

Government of India, 1999, *Bulletin on Rural Health Statistics in India,* Rural Health Division, Directorate General of Health Services, Ministry of Health and family welfare, New Delhi.

Government of India, 2004, *SRS Bulletin*, Registrar General, New Delhi, India, Vol.38, No.1.

Government of India, *National Sample Survey*, 1986-87 and 1995-96.

Government of India, *National Sample Survey*, 57ᵗʰ Round, 'Survey of Unorganised Services', 2001-02.

Government of Tamil Nadu, 1998, *Economic Appraisal, 1997-98,*.

Gubler D.J et al, 2001, 'Climate Variability and Change in the United States: Potential Impacts on Vector- and Rodent- Borne Diseases,' *Environment Health Perspectives*, 109 Suppl. 2.

Gubler DJ, Meltzer M, 1999, 'Impact of Dengue / Dengue Hemorrhagic Fever on the Developing World,' *Adv virus Re*, 53.

Guhan S, 1994, 'Social Security Options for Developing Countries', *International Labour Review*, 133(1).

Halstead S.B, Scanlon J.E, Umpaivit Pand Udomsakdi S, 1969, 'Dengue and Chikungunya Virus in Man in Thailand, 1962-64. IV, Epidemiologic Area,' *American Journal of Tropical Medicine and Hygiene*, 18(6).

Harvey D.A, 2005, *Brief History of Neoliberalism,* Oxford University Press, Oxford.

Hetzel B. S, 1980, *The Story of Iodine Deficiency an International Challenge in Nutrition*, Oxford University Press, Oxford.

Higgs S, 2006, 'The 2005-2006 Chikungunya Epidemic in the India Ocean' *Vector Borne Zoonatic Dis*, 6.

Hodgson T A and Cai L, 2001, 'Medical Care Expenditure for Hypertension, its Complications and its Co Morbidities', *Medical care*, 39(6).

Hodgson T A and Cohen A J, 1999, 'Medical Care Expenditures for Diabetes, its Chronic Complications, and its Co Morbidities', *Preventive Medicine*, 29.

Hodgson T A and Miners M R, 1982, 'Cost of Illness Methodology; A Guide to Current Practices and Procedures', *Milbank memorial fund Quarterly*, 60(3).

Hodgson T A, 1982, 'Annual Cost of Illness Versus Lifetime Costs of Illness and Implications of Structural Change', *Drug Information Journal of Public Health*, 72(6).

Hodgson T A, 1983, 'The State of the Art of Cost of Illness Studies', *Advances in Health Economics and Health Services Research*, 4.

Hodgson T A, 1994, 'Costs of Illness in Cost-Effectiveness Analysis: A Review of the Methodology', *Pharmacoeconomics*, 6(6).

Imrana Qudeer, 2001, *Public Health and the poverty of Nations*, Vikas Publishing House Pvt, Ltd, New Delhi.

Jackson E K, 1995, 'Climate Change and Global infection Disease Threats', *Medical Journal*, Australia, 163.

Jamison D T, 1993, Et al (eds), 'Disease Control Priorities in Developing Countries, Oxford University Press, New York.

Javitz H S, Ward M M, Watson J B, and Jana M, 2004, 'Cost of Illness of Chronic Angina', *The American Journal of Managed Care*, 10(11Suppl).

Jetten. T and Focks D, 1997, 'Potential changes in the Distribution of Dengue Transmission under Climate Warming', *American Journal of Tropical Medicine*, 57.

Jhadhav M, Namboodripad M, Carmen R.H, Carey D.E, Mysers R.M, 1965, 'Chikungunya Disease in Infants and children in Vellore: A Report of Clinical Features of Virollogically Proved Cases', *Indian Journal of Medical Research*, 53.

Johannesson M and Karlsson G, 1996, *Journal of Health Economics,* 16.

John H. Bryant, 1998, 'Health for All: The Dream and the Reality', *Health Action,* P.37.

John T J, 2008, 'Resurgence of Diphtheria in the 21 Century', *Indian Journal of Medical Research*, 128.

John T J, 2009, 'Lessons from the Challenges of Polio Eradication in India', *National Medical Journal of India*, 22.

John T J, Muliyil J, 2009, 'Public Health is Infrastructure for Human Development', *Indian Journal of Medical Research*, 130.

Josseran,L,.C.Paquet, A.zehgnoun,N.Caillere,A. Le Terte, J.solet, and M.Ledrans, 2006 'Chikungunya Disease Outbreak, Reunion Island, Emerging infections Diseases.12:1994.

Juana, J. S.; Narayana, N.; Mupimpila, C., 2004,'Estimating Household Expenditure on Malaria Interventions in Western Sierra Leone: A Contingent Valuation Approach' *International Journal of Environment and Development,* Vol. 1, issue. 1.

Juana, J.S, Narayana N, Mupimpila C, 2004, 'Estimating Household Expenditure on Malaria Interventions in Western Sierra Leone: A Contingent

Kalantri S.P, Joshi R, Riley L.W, 2006, 'Chikungunya Epidemic an Indian Perspective', *National Medical Journal of India*, 19.

Kamali S. S, 1983, Rural *Development and Social change in India*, D.K. Publications, New Delhi.

Kamat S, Das A.K, Parikh F.S, 2006, *Chikungunya*, JAPI, 54.

Karl T.R and Trenbath K, 2003, 'Modern Climate Change', *Science,* 302.

Kawachi I, Wamale S, (eds.), 2007, *Globalization and Health,* Oxford University Press.

Kennedy A.C, Fleming J, and Solomon L, 1980, 'Chikungunya Viral Arthropathy: A Chemical Description,' *J Rheumatol,* 7(2).

Kent, Mary M, Yin Sandra, 2006, 'Controlling Infectious Diseases', *Population Bulletin* Vol.61.issue.2.

Khursed P, 1986, Disappearance of Chikungunya Virus from India and South East Asia,' *Trans Royal Soc Trop Med Hyg,* 80.

Kirshnamoorthy K, Nanda B, Subramanian S, 2008, Chikungunya Emergence inRural South India: Epidemiology- Ogy and Clinical Profile, *Indian Journal of Medical Research.*

Koopmanschap M A and Van Ineveld B M, 1992, 'Towards a New Approach for Estimating Indirect Costs of Disease', *Social Science and Medicine,* 34(9).

Krasovec Katherine and Show Paul R, 2000, 'Reproductive Health and Health Sector Reform Linking Outcome to Action' *The World Bank,* World Bank Institute, Washington D.C., USA.

Krishna M.R, Reddy M.K and Reddy S.R, 2006, Chikungunya Outbreaks in Andrapradesh, *South India current Science,* 91(5).

Kumarasamy V, Pathapa S, Zuridah H, Chem Y.K, Norizah I, Chua K.B, 2006, 'Reemergence of Chikungunya Virus in Malaysia,' *Medical Journal of Malaysia,* 61.

Kurusamy S, 1998, 'Planning for Health', *Social welfare,* Vol.38, No.I.

Lakshmi R. 2003, 'Awareness and Health of Rural woman', *Social Welfare,* vol.4, No.2.

Lam S.K, Chua K.B, Hooi P.S, 2001, 'Chikungunya Infection: Emerging Disease in Malasiya', *Southeast Asian Journal of Tropical Medicine Pus Health,* 32.

Landefeld J S and Seskin E P, 1982, 'The Economic Value of Life: Linking Theory to Practice', *American Journal of Public Health,* 72(6).

Laras K, Sukri N.C, Larasati R.P, Bangs M. J, Kosim R, Djauzi, 2005, 'Tracking the Reemergence of Epidemic Chikungunya Virus in Indonesia', *Trans R soc Tropical Medicine and Hygiene,* 99.

Lazar M.A, 2005, 'How Obesity Causes Diabetes: Not a Fall Tale', *Science,* 307(5708).

Lee K, 'Globalization'in Defels R, Beaglehole R, Lansang M A, Gulliford M (eds.), 2009, *Oxford Textbook of Public Health* (5th edn.) Oxford University Press, Oxford.

Lenglet Y, Barau G. Robillard P.Y, (et al.), 2006, 'Chikungunya Infection in Pregnancy: Evidence for Intrauterine Infection in Pregnant Women and Vertical Transmission in Parturient: Survey of the Reunion Island Outbreak,' *J Gynecol Obstet Biol Ne prods* (Paris), 35(A).

Levin, Simon A, 2007, 'Introduction; Infectious Diseases', *Environment and Development Economics*, Vol.12, Issue, 5.

Lindelow, Magnus, 2005, 'The Utilisation of Curative Healthcare in Mozambique: Does Income Matter?' *Journal of African Economies*, Vol. 14, issue, 3.

Lindelow, Magnus, 2005, 'The Utilization of Curative Healthcare in Mozambique' Does income Matter?' *Journal of African Economies*, Vol.14, Issue, B.

Lingsay S.W and M.H Birky, 1996, 'Climate Change and Malaria Transmission', *Annals of Tropical medicine and Parasitological*, 90(6).

Liu JL, Maniadakis N, Gray A, and Rayner M, 2002, 'The Economic Burden of Coronary Heart Disease in the U K', *Heart*, 88(6).

Lowell B, Schulman G.I, 2005, 'Mitochondrial Dysfunction and Type 2 Diabetes', *Science*, 307(5708).

Luce B.R, Manning W.G, Siegel J.E, and Lipscomb J, 1996, 'Estimating Costs in cost Effectiveness Analysis' in Gold M.R, Siegel J.E, Russell L.B, et al., (eds.), *Cost- effectiveness in Health and medicine*, Oxford University Press, New York.

Lum L.S, Suaya J.A, Lian H.T, San B.K, Sheppard D.S, 2008, 'Quality of Life of Dengue Patients' *American Journal of Tropical Medicine and Hygiene*, 78.

Macroeconomics and Health, November 3, 2001, 'Investing in Health for Economic Development Geneva, *World Health Organization*.

Madiw G, et al, 1997,

'Epidemiology and Treatment of Cyclospora Cayetanensis Infection of Peruvian Children', *Clinical Infectious Diseases*, 24(5).

Mahendradas P, Ranganna S, Shetty R, (et al.), 2008, Ocular Manifestations Associated with Chikungunya', *Ophthalmology*, 115(2).

Malaney Pia, 2003, 'Micro-economic Approaches to Evaluating the Burden of Malaria', *CID working paper*, Harvard, No.99.

Mark T L, Woody G E, Juday T, and Kleber H D, 2001, 'The Economic Costs of Heroin Addiction in the United States', *Drug and Alcohol Dependence*, 61.

Marten P, 1997, 'Health Impacts of Climate Change and Ozone Depletion: An Eco-Epidemiological medaling Approach', 158.

Mathew T, Tiruvengadam K.V, 1973, 'Further Studies on the Isolate of Chikungunya from the Indian Repatriates of Burma', *Indian Journal of Medical Research*, 61 (4).

Mavalankar D, Shastri P, Bandyopadhyay T, Par mar J, Ramani K.V, 2008, 'Increased Mortality Rate Associated with Chikungunya Epidemic, Ahmadabad, India' *Emerging Infectious Disease,* 14(13)

Mavalankar Dileep, Ramani K.V, Jane Show, 2003, 'Management of R H Services in India and the need for Health System Reform' Working Paper, 09-04, *Indian Institute for Management Association.*

Mavalanker D, Shastri P, Ramani K V, 2007, 'Chikungunya Epidemic Mortality in India: Lessons from "17th Century Bills of Mortality Still Relevant, Ahmadabad,' *Indian Institute of Management*, WorkingPaper- No 12:2-12.

Mc Michael A.J, 2001, *Human Frontiers, Environment and Disease: Past Patterns, Future Uncertainties*, Cambridge University Press, Cambridge.

Metha S.R, 1992, *Society and Health,* Vikas Publishing House Pvt. Ltd, New Delhi.

Millennium Ecosystem Assessment, 2005, *Ecosystems and Human well- being, Synthesis Report*, Washington DC, Island Press,

Miller L.S, Zhang X, Novotny T, Rice D.P, and Max W, 1998, 'State Estimates of Medicaid Expenditures Attributable to cigarette Smoking', Fiscal year 1993, *Public Health Reports*, 113(2).

Mishan E J, 1971, 'Evaluation of Life and Limb: A Theoretical Approach', Journal of Political Economy, 79(4).

Mishra B, Ratho R.K, 2006, 'Chikungunya Reemergence: Possible Mechanism,' *Lancet,* 368.

Mohan A, 2006, 'Chikungunya Fever: Clinical Manifestation and Management,' *India J med Res,* No.124.Mohan A, 2006, 'Chikungunya Fever: Clinical Manifestations and Management', *Indian Journal of Medical Research*, 124.

Morganstern H, Klein Baum D G, and Kupper L L, 1980, 'Measures of Diseases Incidence Used in Epidemiological Research', *International Journal of Epidemiology*, 9.

Mourya D.T, Mishra A. C, 2006, 'Chikungunya Fever', *Lancet*, Vol.368.

Mourya D.T, 1987, 'Absense of Transovarial Transmission of Chikungunya Virus in Aedes aegypti and Ae. Albopictus', *Indian Journal of Medical Research,* 85.

Musgrove, Philip, ed., 2004, *Health economics in development'.*

Nakicenovic N, and R.J Swart, (eds.), 2001, *IPCC Special Report on Emissions Scenarios*, Cambridge University Press, Cambridge.

National Institute of Communicable Disease, 2006, Chikungunya Fever CD Alert 10, New Delhi, (2).

Neogi D.K, Bhatta Charya N, Mukherjee K.K, (et al),2006, 'Sero Survey of Chikungunya Antibody in Calcutta Metropolis,' *J Commun Dis*, 1995,37.

Nicholls N, 1994, 'EI Nino –Southern Oscillation and Vector bone Disease', in *Health and climate change*, (ed.), D. Sharp, Lancet.

Outbreak New, 'Chikungunya and Dengue South –West India Ocean', *Weekly Epidemic Record*, 2006, 81.

Padbidri V.S, Gnaneswar T.T, 1979, 'Epidemiological Investigation of Chikungunya Epidemic at Barsi- Maharashtra State, India', *Journal of Hygienic Epidemiology Microbial Immunology*, 23(4).

Padbidri V.S,Gnaneswar T.T, 1979, 'Epidemiological Investigations of Chikungunya Epidemic at Barsi', *Microbial Manual*, 23.

Pagano E, Brunetti M, Tediosi F, and Garattini L,1999, 'Costs of Diabetes: A Methodological Analysis of the Literature' *Pharmacoeconomics*, 15(6).

PAHO, 1982, 'Epidemiologic Disease Surveillance after Disaster', *Scientific Publication*, 420, pp. 3-4, and 'Emergency Vector Control after Natural Disaster', *Scientific Publication*, 419.

Panicker, K.N. & Rajagopalan, P.K. 1986, 'Vector Control through Integrated Rural Development', *ICMR Bulletin*, Vol.16, No.1.

Parik, 1986, 'Disappearance of Chikungunya Virus from India and Southern Asia,' *Trans R Soc Trop med Hyg*; 80.

Park J.E. and Park.K, 1983, 'Health Care of the Community', *Text Book of Preventive and Social Medicine*, Banarsidas, Jabalpur.

Park K. Parks, 2005, *Text book of Preventive and Social Medicine*, in Bhanot B.D, editor. 18th ed. Jabalpur.

Parvi K, 1986, 'Disappearance of Chikungunya Virus from Indian and Southeast Asia', *Trans R Soc Tropical Med Hygiene*, 80.

Pialoux G, Gauzere B. A, Jaureguiberrys, Straubel M, 2007, 'Chikungunya An Epidemic Arbovirosis, *Lancet Infect Dis*, Issues (5).

Pialoux G, Gauzere B.A, Jaureguiberry S, Strobel M, 2007, 'Chikungunya, an Epidemic Arbovirosis,' *Lancet infect Dis*, 7(5).

Pialoux G, Gauzere B.A, Jaurequiberry S and Stobel M, 2007, 'Review: Chikungunya an Epidemic Arbovirosis, *Lancet infect Dis*, 7.

Population Reference Bureau, 2004, *Improving the Health of the World's Poorest People*, Policy Brief, Washington D.C.

Powers AM, Logue CH, 2007, 'Changing Patterns of Chikungunya Virus: Re-emergence of a Zoonotic Arbovirus,' *Journal of Genetic Virology*, 88.

Powersa M, Broulta C, Tesh R.B, Weaver S.C, 2000, 'Reemergence of Chickungunya and Onyongnuong Viruses: Evidences for districts', *Geographical Lineages and Districts Evolutionary Relationships Environ*, 81.

Rameshwaran G, 1989, *Medical and Health Administration in Rural India,* Ashish Publishing House, New Delhi, P.18.

Ramful D, Carbonnier M, Pasquet,(et. al), 2007, 'Mother-to-child Transmission of Chikungunya Virus Infections', *Prediator Infect Dis Journal,* 26 (9).

Rao R Sujatha, 2004, 'Health Insurance Concepts, Issues and challenges,' *Economics and Political Weekly*, August 21.

Ratnasamy Prabhavati, 2000, 'Health Care is a Right Not Privilege', *Social Welfare*, Vol.47, No.1.

Ravi V, 2006, 'Re-emergence of Chikungunya Virus in India', *Indian Journal of Medical Microbiology*, 24.

Reddy K S, Shah B, Varghese C, Ramada's A, 2005, 'Responding to the Threat of Chronic Diseases in India', *Lancet*, 366.

Reynaud M, Gaudin-Colombel AN F, and Le Pen C, 2001, 'Two Methods of Estimating Health Costs Linked to Alcoholism in France (With a Note on Social Costs)', *Alcohol and Alcoholism,* 36(1).

Rice D P, 1967, 'Estimating the Cost of Illness American Journal of Public Health, 57(3.).

Rice D P, 2000, 'Cost of illness Studies: What is Good about Them?' *Injury Prevention*, 6.

Rice D P, Fox P J, Max W, Webber P A, Lindeman D A, Hauck W, and Segura E, 1993, 'The Economic Burden of Alzheimer's Disease Care', *Health Affairs*, 12(2).

Rice D P, Kelman S, Miller L S, and Dunmeyer S,1990, 'The Economic Costs of Alcohol and Drug Abuse and Mental Illness', 1985, Rockville, M D: *National institute on Drug Abuse*.

Rice D, 1999, The Economic Burden of Musculoskeletal Conditions, U S, 1995, in Praemer A, Furner S, and Rice D.P (eds), Musculoskeletal Condition in the U S Rosemont, I.L, *American Academy of Orthopedic Surgeons.*

Rice D.P, Mackenzie E.J, 1989, 'Associate Cost of Injury in the United States: A Report to Congress, San Francisco, *C A: Institute for Health and Aging*, Johns Hopkins University.

Roberts, Jennifer A., ed., 2006, *'The Economic of Infectious Disease'*.

Robinson M.C, 1955, 'An Epidemic of Virus Disease in Southern Province, Tanganjika Territory, in 1952-53, Clinical Features' *Trans R Soc Trop Med Hyg*, 49.

Rockhill B, Newman B, and Weinberg C, 1998, 'Use and Misuse of Population Attributable Fractions', *American Journal of Public Health*, 88(1).

Rogowski J, 1999, 'Measuring the Cost of Prenatal and Parental care', *Pediatrics*, 103(suppl 1 E).

Ross RW, 1956, 'The Newalla epidemic 111; The Virus: Isolation, Pathogenic properties and relationship to the epidemic', *Journal of Hygiene*, 54.

Rothermich EA and Pathak D S, 1999, 'Productivity Cost Controversies in Cost-Effectiveness Analysis: Review and Research Agenda', *Clinical Therapeutics*, 21(1).

Roux L and Donaldson C, 2004, 'Economics and Obesity: Costing the Problems or Evaluating Solutions?', *Obesity Research*, 12.

Sach S J, Warner A, 1995, 'Economic Reform and the Process of Global Integration Brookings Papers', *Econ Activity*, 1.

Sachs J, Malancy P, 2002, 'The Economic and Social Burden of Malaria', *Nature,* 415.

Sachs J.D, 2005, *The End of Poverty: Economic Possibilities for Our Time*, Penguin, New York.

Salazar- Lindo E, Pinell-Salles P, Marcy A, and Chea- woo E, 1997, 'EI Nino and Diarrhoea and Dehydration in Lima, Peru', *Lancet*, 350 (9091).

Santer and Near, 1960, *Health Economics*, Irwin Publication, London.

Santerr and Neun, 1996, *Health Economics*, Irwin Publication, London.

Saxena S.K. Singh M, Mishra N, Lakshmi V, 2006, 'Resurgence of Chikungunya Virus in India: An Emerging Threat', *Euro surveill*, 11:E060810.2.

Schieber G, maeda A, 1997, 'Curmudgeon's Guide to Health Care Financing in Developing Countries, Schieber G, editor, 'Innovations in health care financing', Washington (DC), World Bank 1997, 'Proceedings of a World Bank Conference', 10-11 march.

Schuffenecker I, Iteman I, Michault A, Murris, Frangeul L, Vaney MC,2006, (et. al), 'Genome Microevolution of Chikungunya Viruses Causing the Indian Ocean outbreak, *PLOS Med,* 3.

Seul S.L, 1975, *Health Administration in India*, Dawn Books, Calcutta.

Shangar Uma and Misra Girish K, (ed) 1993,*Urban health System*, Reliance Publishing House, New Delhi.

Sharp, Ansel M and Register, Charles A, 1987, *Economics of Social Issues,* Universal Book Stall, New Delhi.

Shaw K.V. Gibbs C.J. Jr & Banerjee G. 1964, 'Virological Investigation of Epidemic of Haemorhagic Fever in Calcutta – Isolation of Three Chikungunya Virus', *Indian Journal of Medical Research,* Vol. 52.

Shepard D.S., Ettling, M.B., Brinkmann, U & Sauerborn, R. 1991, 'The Economic Cost of Malaria in Africa', *Tropical Medicine and Parasitology,* Vol.42, No.3.

Simon F, Parole P, Granddame M, (et al.), 2007, 'Chikungunya Infection: An Emerging Rheumatism among Travelers Returned from Indian Ocean Islands, Report of 47 Cases', *Medicine* (Baltimore), 86(3).

Singh K.V, Parvi K.M, 1967, 'Experimental Studies with Chikungunya Virus in Aedes aegypti and Aedes albopictus', *Acta Virol,* 11.

Singh N, Shukla M.M, Mishra A.K, Singh M. P, Pailwal J.C, Dash A. P, 2006, 'Malaria Control Using Indoor Residual Sprajing and Carnivorous Fish: A Case study in Betel, Central India', *Tropical Medicine Internal Health,* 11.

Staikowsky F, Pinar A, Land E, Grivard P, Tallermin F, Michauld A, 2006, 'The Infection by the Virus Chikungunya; An Emergent Disease in the Reunion Island,' *Eur J Emerg med,*13: A.

Stine R, 1995, 'Global warming if the Mercury Soars, So may Health Hazards'. News and Comments, *Science,* 267.

Swaroop A, Jain A, Kumar M, Parihar N, and Jain S, 2007, Review Article, 'Chikungunya Fever', *Indian Academy of clinical medicine,*8(2).

Taylor D.H, and Sloan F.A, 2000, 'How Much Do Persons with Alzheimer's Disease Cost Medicare?,' *Journal of the American Geriatrics Society,* 48.

Thaikruea L, Charearnsook O, Reanphum Karnkit S, Dissomboon P, Phonjan R, Ratchbud S, (et al) 1997, 'Chikungunya in Thailand A Reemerging Disease,' *South East Asian Journal of Tropical Medicine and Public Health,* 28.

Thaper S. T, 1977, *Health and Development,* Association of Voluntary Agencies for Rural Development, New Delhi.

The Hindu, 1999, 'Major Health Care Scheme for Poor', *The Hindu* Daily, 9 Nov.

The World Health Report, 2000, 'Health Systems: Measuring Performance Geneva', World Health organization.

Thiruvengadam K.V, Kalyanasundaram V, Rajagopal J, 1965, 'Clinical and Pathological Studies in Chikungunya Fever in Madras City', *Indian Journal of Medical Research*, 53.

Thompson D, Edelsberg J, Kinsey K.L, Oster G,1998, 'Estimated Economic Costs of Obesity to US Businesses', *American Journal of Health Promotion*,13(2).

Umashankar P.K and Girish K. Misra (ed), 1993, *Urban Health System*, Reliance Publishing House, New Delhi.

Valuation Approach,' *Journal of International Environment and Development*, Vol-1, Issue 1.

Van Ginneken W, 1999, 'Social Security for the Informal Sector: New challenges for the developing Countries', *International Social Security Review*, 52(1.

Verma K.K, 1992, *Health Care and Family Welfare*, Mittal Publications, New Delhi.

Visaria L, 2000, 'Innovations in Tamil Nadu', Presented at a Symposium on *The State of our Public Health System*.

Vishwakarma R.K, 1993, *Health Status of the Under Privileged*, Reliance Publishing House, New Delhi.

Wadia R.S, 2007, Presidential Oration: A Neurotropic Virus (Chikungunya) and a Neurotropic Amino acid (homocysteine)', *Ann India head neurol*, 10.

Warner K.E, Flodgson T.A, and Carroll C.E, 1999, 'Medical Costs of Smoking in the United States: Estimates, Their Validity and Their implication', *Tobacco Control*, 8.

Weiss R.A and Michael A. J, 2004, 'Social and Environmental Risk Factors in the Emergence of Infectious Diseases', *Nature med*, 10.

WHO- SEARO, 2007, Communicable Diseases, *Newsletter*, 4(3) pp.1-5.

Wilder Smith A, Schwartz E, 2005, 'Dengue in Travelers', *N English Journal of Medicine*, 353.

Wilson M L, 2001, 'Ecology and Infections disease' in *Ecosystem Change and Public Health: A Global Perspective*, Aron J.L. and Patz, J.A, (eds.), John Hopkins University Press, Baltimore, USA.

World Bank, 1993, *World Development Report 1993*, 'Investing in Health', Oxford University Press, New York.

World Bank, 1997, *The State in a Changing World; World Development Report 1997*, Oxford University Press, Oxford.

World Health Organisation, 2000, International Conference on Mosquito Control: Recommendations, *Weekly Epidemic Research 2000*, WHO, 75.

World Health Organization - South- East Asia Regional Office, 2008, 'Chikungunya in South East Asia update'.

World Health Organization, 2007, 'Outbreak and Spread of Chikungunya,' Weakly Epidemiological Records, 82 (47).

Yergollcar P, Tandale B, Arankalle V, (et al), 2006, 'Chikungunya outbreaks caused by African genotype, India', *Emerge in fact Dis,* 12.

Zaidi A.K.M, Awasthi S, Desilva H.J, 2004, 'Burden of Infection Diseases in South Asia,' *Bangladesh Medical Journal*, 328.

Zeller M, Sharma M, 2005. 'Many Borrow, More Save, and all Insure: Implications for Food and Micro- Finance Policy, *Food Policy,* 25(2).

Zytoon E.M, El-Belbasi H.I, Matsumura T,1993 'Mechanism of Increased Dissemination of Chikungunya Virus in Aedes albopictus Mosquitoes Concurrently Ingesting Microfilariae of Dirofilaria Immitis' *American Journal of Tropical Medicine and Hygiene*, 49.

Appendix-Questionnaire

The Economic Impact Of Chikungunya Fever
On Household Level In Tamil Nadu: A Study
In Kanayakumari District

A. IDENTIFICATION PARTICULARS

A. 1. Name of the respondent :
A. 2. Address :
A. 3. Area :1.Vilavancode, 2.Kalkulam

B. HOUSEHOLD PARTICULARS
(To be addressed to the head of the household)

B. 1. Sex : 1. Male   2. Female
B. 2. Age : ——————— Years
B. 3. Caste: ———————————
B. 4. Community

    1. Schedule Caste   2. Scheduled Tribe
    3. Most Backward Class 4. Backward Class
    5. Others ———— (Specify)

B. 5. Religion

    1. Hindu   2. Christian
    3. Muslim   4. Others———— (Specify)

B. 6. Mother Tongue

    1. Tamil   2. Telugu

    3. Malayalam   4. Kannada

    5. Hindi   6. Others _____ (Specify)

B. 7. Marital Status

    1. Unmarried   2. Married

    3. Widow/Widower   4. Divorced/Separated

B. 8. Literacy Status

    1. Literate   2. Illiterate

B. 9. Educational Standard

    1. Primary School   2. Middle School

    3. High School   4. Higher Secondary

    5. Graduates   6. Post-Graduates

    7. Professionals   8. Others _____ (Specify)

B. 10. Type of Family

    1. Nuclear   2. Joint   3. Uni-Member

B. 11. Occupation   _____

C. HOUSEHOLD COMPOSITION

Sl. No	Name	Relationship with the head	Age	Sex	Literacy Standard	Marital Status	Activity Status	Occupation	Monthly Income (in Rs)	Chikungunya Affected
1		Self								
2										
3										
4										
5										
6										
7										
8										

C. 1. Household size (nos): _____

C. 2. Number on male members: _____

C. 3. Number of female members: _____

C. 4. Total number of male children (below 15 years): _____

C. 5. Total number of female children (below 15 years): _____

C. 6. Number of school going male children at the school going age (5 years – below 15 years): _____

C. 7. Number of school going female children at the school Going age (5 years – below 15 years): _____

C. 8. Number of working aged male members (Between 15 and 60 years): _____

C. 9. Number of working aged female members: _____

C. 10. Number of male employed in the working age: _____

C. 11. Number of female employed in the working age: _____

C. 12. Number of aged male workers (above 60 years): _____

C. 13. Number of aged female workers (above 60 years): _____

C. 14. Number of illiterate male: _____

C. 15. Number of illiterate female: _____

C. 16. Number of married male: _____

C. 17. Number of married female: _____
C. 18. Number of male income earners: _____
C. 19. Number of female income earners: _____

D. ECONOMIC BACKGROUND

D. 1. Income of the respondent: Rs._____
D. 2. Income earned by other family members: Rs._____
D. 3. Income from other sources: Rs._____
D. 4. Total monthly household income: Rs._____
D. 5. (a). Expenditure on food taken outside home:

    Daily Rs_____ Weekly Rs_____
    Monthly Rs_____

D. 5. (b). Expenditure on preparing food per day:

    Daily Rs_____ Weekly Rs_____
    Monthly Rs_____

D. 5. (c). Total monthly expenditure on food: Rs._____
D. 5. (d). Monthly expenditure on fuel/electricity: Rs._____
D. 5. (e). Clothing: Rs. _____
D. 5. (f). Rent/annual maintenance of house:Rs. _____
D. 5. (g). Education: Rs. _____
D. 5. (h). Entertainment: Rs. _____
D. 5. (i). Transportation: Rs. _____
D.5. (j). Habits (smoking, chewing/others): Rs. _____
D. 5. (k). Festivals and ceremonies: Rs. _____
D. 5. (l). Medicines/consultation: Rs. _____
D. 5. (m). Dept repayment: Rs. _____
D. 5. (n). Chits: Rs. _____
D. 5. (o). others _____ Specify: Rs. _____
D. 6. Total average monthly household expenditure: Rs. _____
D. 7. Do you have any savings at present?

    1. Yes   2. No

D. 8. If yes, what is your current savings?: Rs. _____
D. 9. Are you a debtor?

    1. Yes   2. No

D. 10. If yes, what is the total outstanding debt at present?:
       Rs. _____
D. 11. What is the approximate value of your wealth at present?:
       Rs. _____

E. HOUSING

E. 1. What is the nature of tenancy of your residence?

    1. Owned   2. Rented   3. Leased

E. 2. Is your house electrified?

    1. Yes   2. No

E. 3. Approximate area of the house: _____ sq.ft
E. 4. What is the nature of your house?

    1. Concrete   2. Tiled
    3. Roof made up of coconut leaves
    4. Roof made up on hay/straws
    5. Others _____ (specify)

E. 5. Specify the number of windows in your house: _____
E. 6. Specify the number of rooms in your house: _____
E. 7. What is the nature of access way to the house?

    1. Vehicular Road   2. Paved Path
    3. Unpaved Path   4. Others _____ (specify)

E. 8. What is the distance of your house to the vehicular path?:
       _____ mts

F. SANITATION

F. 1. Is there any water stagnating area near your residence?

1. Yes   2. No

F. 2. What is the source of drinking water?

1. Open Well   2. Bore Well   3. Public tap
4. Others _____ (specify)

F. 3. Where do you store water for day-to-day use?

1. Overhead tank   2. Pots
3. Open storage tank 4. Others _____ (specify)

F. 4. If you have an overhead tank in your house, is it kept open?

1. Yes   2. No

F. 5. Where do you dispose waste coconut shell, cycle tube and vessels?

1. In the backyard   2. In the disposal site

F. 6. Is there any open area near your residence?

1. Yes   2. No

F. 7. Do you have toilet facility in your house?

1. Yes   2. No

F. 8. Do you rear cattle or any other animal at your home?

1. Yes   2. No

HEALTH PROBLEMS DUE TO CHIKUNGUNYA FEVER

G. 1. How many members of your family did suffer from Chikungunya fever in the last year?: _____

G. 2. Age composition of Chikungunya affected members

	MALE	FEMALE	TOTAL
Children less than 5 years			
Children aged between 5 and 15 years			
Aged between 15 and 60 years			
Aged 60 years and above			
Total			

G. 3. Is there any pregnant women in your family affected by Chikungunya fever?

1. Yes   2. No

G. 4. If yes, was there any problem at the time of child birth?

1. Yes   2. No

G. 5. What is the nature of Chikungunya infection in your household?

1. All family members were affected by Chikungunya at a time
2. All of the family members were affected simultaneously
3. Some of the members were affected at a time
4. Some of the members were affected simultaneously
5. Some of the members were affected in different periods in a year

G. 6. How did you come to know that the fever is Chikungunya?

	P₁	P₂	P₃	P₄	P₅	P₆
Laboratory examination						
Clinical symptoms						
Doctor's diagnosis						
Others						

G. 7. Was there any wage earner affected due to Chikungunya fever?

     1. Yes   2. No

G. 8. If yes, how many? _____

G. 9. How did you manage expenses related to medical care?

     1. From the past   2. Borrowed money
        savings
     3. Support from friends and relatives
     4. Depend on public health centres
     5. Others _____ (Specify)

G. 10. Answer the level of the following questions which are related to the level of sickness of Chikungunya fever.

	P₁	P₂	P₃	P₄	P₅	P₆
Pain						
Suffering						
Worrying being about the victims						

Code: 1. Mild, 2. Moderate, 3. Severe

G. 11. What are the symptoms of Chikungunya fever occurred for you?

SYMPTOMS	P_1	P_2	P_3	P_4	P_5	P_6
1.Sudden fever						
2. Cough						
3. Swelling						
4. Chills						
5. Headache						
6. Nausea						
7. Vomiting						
8. Joint Pain						
9. Rash						
10. Abdominal Pain						

1. Present   0. Absent

G. 12. Details of sick persons

DETAILS	P_1	P_2	P_3	P_4	P_5	P_6
Age(in years)						
Sex*						
Marital Status						
Source of medical assistance**						

Code: *1. Male   2. Female

     **1. Private   2. Public   3. Both

G. 13. Type of treatment given to the sick persons

TREATMENT	P_1	P_2	P_3	P_4	P_5	P_6
1. Allopathy*						
2. Homeopathy*						
3. Sidha*						
4. Ayurveda*						
5. Unani*						
6. Others*						
13. Why did you select this treatment?						

Code:* 1. Yes   2. No
    ** 1. It cures better than any other treatment
       2. Most of the neighbours select this particular source
       3. Don't have money to choose other sources
       4. Others _____ (Specify)

G. 14. Are you suffering from:

NON-INFECTIOUS DISEASES	P_1	P_2	P_3	P_4	P_5	P_6
1. Blood pressure						
2. Diabetes						
3. Ulcer						
4. Arthritis						
5. Cancer						
6. Tuberculosis						

     1. Yes   0. No

	P_1	P_2	P_3	P_4	P_5	P_6
15. Did you face the problem of sleeplessness during the fever?						
16. Whether Chikungunya fever occurred to you before?						
17. Did you consult doctor for treating Chikungunya Fever?						
18. Did any one of the sick persons experience complication as a result of taking treatment?						

     Code: 1. Yes   2. No

G. 19. When did you consult doctor for treating Chikungunya Fever?

	P_1	P_2	P_3	P_4	P_5	P_6
Time of Treatment*						
Duration of sickness (Days)						

     Code*:1. As soon as felt the symptom of disease
         2. When fever did not allow performing work
         3. Taken treatment when it became very serious

G. 20. If treated when fever became serious, what was the reason for the late medical care?

	P_1	P_2	P_3	P_4	P_5	P_6
Reason for the late medical care*						

Code:*1. Clinics and hospitals far away from residence
    2. Over crowdedness in hospitals
    3. Cannot afford
    4. No one to take to hospital
    5. Others _____ (specify)

G. 21. How many days it took to recover from fever? _____ days
G. 22. After recovering from fever, how many days it took to bring you back to the normal health situation? _____ days
G. 23. How long you have been suffering from the illness due to Chikungunya? _____
G. 24. How long have you been suffering the side effects due to Chikungunya fever? _____
G. 25. Can you be able to take the same workload after recovering from the Chikungunya Fever?

1. Yes   2. No   ☐

G. 26. If no, did you change the occupation after recovering from the fever?

1. Yes   2. No   ☐

G. 26. Out patients

DIRECT COST	P_1	P_2	P_3	P_4
Number of doctors visits				
Number of working days lost due to Chikungunya Fever				
Doctors fee for each consultation (Rs)				
Cost of diagnostic tests (Rs)				
Cost of medicines (Rs)				

Cost of transportation (Rs)				
Number of persons accompanied with you in every visit				
Cost of transportation between residence and hospital (Rs)				
Did you face any problem in getting admission to indoor treatment in hospital?				

Code: 1. Yes   0. No

G. 27. If yes, why? _____

	P_1	P_2	P_3	P_4	P_5	P_6
Doctors fee per admission(Rs)						
Diagnostic tests(Rs)						
Number of days stayed in the hospital						
Accommodation cost(Rs)						
Transport cost(Rs)						
Wage loss to the sick person(Rs)						
Wage loss to the bystander(Rs)						
Was there any death in your family due to Chikungunya*?						
If yes, the age of the diseased person(years)						

*Code: 1. Yes   2. No

H. AFTERMATH EFFECT

H.1. Are you suffer from after-effects of Chikungunya?

1. Yes   2. No

H.2. Did you lose any working day?

1. Yes   2. No

H.3. If yes, how many days? _____

H.4. What is the approximate wage loss after the Chikungunya fever recovery? Rs. _____

H.5. Do you have the same acceptance from the employer after Chikungunya?

1. Yes   2. No   ☐

H.6. Did you face the following problems to your family as a result of Chikungunya Fever?

PROBLEMS	P_1	P_2	P_3	P_4	P_5	P_6
Dropping of school attendance						
Absenteeism in work after recovery						
Marriage postponed						
Festivals not celebrated						
Exploitation by clinics and hospitals						

1. Yes   0. No

I. PERCEPTIONS

I. 1. Is Chikungunya an infectious disease?

1. Yes   2. No   ☐

I. 2. Chikungunya is transmitted by

1. Mosquito bite   2. Houseflies bite   ☐
3. Drinking of polluted water   4. Spread through air
5. Due to sins   6. No idea
7. Others _____ (Specify)

I. 3. How important is the clean environment for you?

1. Very important   2. Important   3. Not important   ☐

I. 4. Did anybody advise you how to prevent Chikungunya Fever?

1. Yes   2. No   ☐

I. 5. If yes, what were there advices?

1. _____
2. _____
3. _____
4. _____
5. _____

I. 6. Preventive measures

1. Mosquito coil   2. Bed nets
3. Mosquito liquid repellent   4. Others _____ (Specify)

I. 7. Did anybody suggest you to isolate the sick person from other person to avoid transmission to others?

1. Yes   2. No

I. 8. What do you think for the cause of the fever?

Appendix-II

Glossary

Alpha virus	-	genus of single-stranded RNA viruses of the family *Togaviridae* that are transmitted by arthropods and especially mosquitoes and that include the Mayaro virus, Semliki Forest virus, Sindbis virus, and the causative agents of chikungunya and equine encephalitis.
Analgesic	-	Relating to, characterized by, or producing analgesia.
Anopheles	-	A genus of mosquitoes that includes all mosquitoes that transmit malaria to humans.
Anorexia	-	Loss of appetite especially when prolonged.
Anthropogenesis	-	The origin and development of humans.
Antigenemia	-	The condition of having an antigen in the blood.
Arthritis	-	Inflammation of joints due to infectious, metabolic, or constitutional causes.
Arthropathy	-	A disease of a joint.
Asymmetrical	-	Bonded to four different atoms or groups: not symmetrical.
Capillary	-	**Resembling** a hair especially in slender elongated form having a very small bore.
Capsid	-	The protein shell of a virus particle that surrounds its nucleic acid.
Catastrophic	-	of an illness: financially ruinous: of, relating to, resembling, or resulting in catastrophe.
Chronological age	-	The age of a person as measured from birth to a given date.

Conjunctiva	-	The mucous membrane that lines the inner surface of the eyelids and is continued over the forepart of the eyeball.
Diagnosis	-	The art or act of identifying a disease from its signs and symptoms.
Dimorphous	-	Crystallizing in two different forms.
Dyschromia	-	Abnormal pigmentation of the skin <periocular*dyschromia*.
Echymosis	-	The escape of blood into the tissues from ruptured blood vessels marked by a livid black-and-blue or purple spot o area; *also*: the discoloration so caused.
Epidemiology	-	A branch of medical science that deals with the incidence, distribution, and control of disease in a population.
Erythema	-	Abnormal redness of the skin due to capillary congestion (as in inflammation).
Etiologic	-	Branch of medical science dealing with the causes an origin of diseases.
Genome	-	one haploid set of chromosomes with the genes they contain.
Genotype	-	All or part of the genetic constitution of an individual or group.
Hemorrhage	-	A copious discharge of blood from the blood vessels.
Hemorrhagic dengue	-	any of a diverse group of virus diseases (as Korean hemorrhagic fever, Lassa fever, and Ebola) that are usually transmitted to humans by arthropods or rodents and are characterized by a sudden onset, fever, aching, bleeding in the internal organs (as of the gastrointestinal tract), petechiae, and shock.
Hyperpigmentation	-	Excess pigmentation in a bodily part or tissue (as the skin).
Icosahedra capsid	-	protein shell of a virus.
Kinematic viscosity	-	The ratio of the coefficient of viscosity to the density of a fluid.

Leucopoenia – A condition in which the number of white blood cells circulating in the blood is abnormally low and which is most commonly due to a decreased production of new cells in conjunction with various infectious diseases, as a reaction to various drugs or other chemicals, or in response to irradiation.

Lichenoid - Resembling lichen <a *lichenoid* eruption> <*lichenoid* dermatitis>

Lymphadenopathy - Abnormal enlargement of the lymph nodes.

lymphedema - Edema due to faulty lymphatic drainage.

Maculopapular - combining the characteristics of macules and papules <a *maculopapular* rash>.

Meningoencephalitis - Inflammation of the brain and meninges— called also *encephalomeningitis*.

Myalgia - Pain in one or more muscles.

Nausea - A stomach distress with distaste for food and an urge to vomit.

Neonatal - Affecting the newborn and especially the human infant during the first month after birth.

Nucleotide - any of several compounds that consist of a ribose or deoxyribose sugar joined to a purine or pyramiding base and to a phosphate group and that are the basic structural units of RNA and DNA— compare.

Paracetamol - A crystalline compound $C_8H_9NO_2$ that is a hydroxyl derivative of acetanilide and is used in chemical synthesis and in medicine instead of aspirin to relieve pain and fever.

Pathogen - A specific causative agent (as a bacterium or virus) of disease.

Peplomer - Glycoprotein spike on a viral capsid or viral envelope.

Pharyngitis - Inflammation of the pharynx.

Phospholipids   -   any of numerous lipids (as lecithin's and phosphatidylethanolamines) in which phosphoric acid as well as a fatty acid is esterifies to glycerol and which are found in all living cells and in the bilayers of cell membranes—called also *phosphatide*, *phospholipin*.

Photophobia   -   intolerance to light; *especially*: painful sensitiveness to strong light: an abnormal fear of light.

Phylogenetic   -   Off or relating to phylogeny: based on natural evolutionary relationships: acquired in the course of phylogenetic development.

Pigmentary   -   of, relating to, or containing pigment.

Polyarthritis   -   Arthritis involving two or more joints.

Polyarthritis   -   Arthritis involving two or more joints.

Polymerase   -   Any of several enzymes that catalyze the formation of DNA or RNA from precursor substances in the presence of pre-existing DNA or RNA acting as a template.

Polyneuritis   -   Neuritis of several peripheral nerves at the same time (as that caused by vitamin B deficiency, a toxic substance, or an infectious disease.

Sindbis virus   -   a togavirus of the genus *Alphavirus* (species *Sindbis virus*) that is transmitted by mosquitoes and causes a febrile disease marked by joint pain, a rash, and malaise in parts of Africa, the Middle East, Europe, Asia, and Australia.

Stephanurus   -   Genus of nematode worms of the family Strongylidae that includes the kidney worm (*S. dentatus*) of swine.

Subungual   -   situated or occurring under a fingernail or toenail <a *subungual* abscess>.

Sylvatic plague - A form of plague of which wild rodents and their fleas are the reservoirs and vectors and which is widely distributed in western North and South America though rarely affecting humans.T

Tenosynovitis - Inflammation of a tendon sheath— called also *tendovaginitis, tenovaginitis.*

Thrombocytopenia - Persistent decrease in the number of blood platelets that is often associated with hemorrhagic conditions—called also *thrombopenia.*

Togaviridae - a family of single-stranded RNA viruses that have a spherical virion about 70 nanometres' in diameter and that include the causative agents of German measlesand the three equine encephalomyelitide.

Togaviridae - A family of single-stranded RNA viruses that have a spherical virion about 70 manometers in diameter and that include the causative agents of German measles and the three equine encephalomyelitides.

Transovarial - Relating to or being transmission of a pathogen from an organism (as a tick) to its offspring by infection of eggs in its ovary.

Urticaria - An allergic disorder marked by raised oedematous red patches of skin or mucous membrane and usually by intense itching and caused by contact with a specific precipitating factor (as a food, drug, or inhalant) either externally or internally.

Vertebrate - Having a spinal column.

Vesiculobullous - of, relating to, or being both vesicles and bullae <a *vesiculobullous* rash>.

Viremia - The presence of viruses in the blood.

Virology - A branch of science that deals with viruses.

Vitellus - The egg cell proper including the yolk but excluding any albuminous or membranous envelopes.

www.ingramcontent.com/pod-product-compliance
Lightning Source LLC
Chambersburg PA
CBHW030424290526
45786CB00001B/128